Comprehensive and Clinical Anatomy of the Middle Ear

Salah Mansour • Jacques Magnan
Hassan Haidar • Karen Nicolas
Stéphane Louryan

Comprehensive and Clinical Anatomy of the Middle Ear

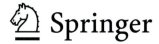 Springer

Authors

Salah Mansour, MD, FRCSC
Lebanese University
Hospital Sacre Coeur
ORL Chirurgie Cervico - Faciale
Baabda
Lebanon

Hôpital Trad
ORL Chirurgie Cervico - Faciale
Beirut
Lebanon

Jacques Magnan, MD, PhD
University Aix-Marseille
Hôpital Nord
ORL - Chirurgie Cervico - Faciale
Marseille
France

Hassan Haidar, MD, ABORL
Hôpital Nord
ORL - Chirurgie Cervico - Faciale
Marseille
France

Karen Nicolas, MD
Department of Radiology
Lebanese University
Middle East Institute of Health, Bsalim
Levant Clinics
Beirut
Lebanon

Department of Radiology
Levant Clinics
Sinn el Fil
Lebanon

Stéphane Louryan, MD, PhD
Laboratoire d`Anatomie
Biomécanique et Organogenèse
Université Libre de Bruxelles
Faculté de Médecine
Brussels
Belgium

ISBN 978-3-642-36966-7   ISBN 978-3-642-36967-4   (eBook)
DOI 10.1007/978-3-642-36967-4
Springer Heidelberg New York Dordrecht London

Library of Congress Control Number: 2013943470

Printed on acid-free paper

Springer is part of Springer Science+Business Media (www.springer.com)

To my wife Ruth: my life's projects would not have been possible without her love and support.
Also to my three sons, Jana, Ryhan, and Fady: they made me proud.

Salah Mansour

Preface

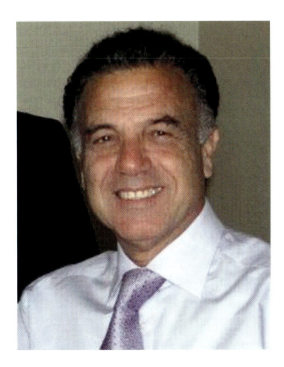

Otology and clinical achievements in dealing with middle ear diseases have historically relied on the valuable work of anatomists, beginning with the Renaissance and throughout the revolutionary era of temporal bone microscopic dissections. During the last 20 years, thanks to the advanced work and research of otologists, new knowledge of middle ear anatomy had great impact on the understanding of middle ear functions, the management of pathologies, and applicable rehabilitation measures.

Most otolaryngology and otology textbooks have however continued to describe the anatomy and embryology of the middle ear with limited detail, thus inadequately serving the needs of learners. Candidates have long emphasized the need for a single, organized volume covering the latest developments in sufficient detail.

Our work is an integrated teaching tool and a source of reference to the available specialty literature. The authors' purpose is to offer complete, up-to-date coverage of the anatomy of the middle ear, so as to enable those undergoing surgical training to find and understand both essential and advanced information, and orient clinical decisions and surgical approaches.

This book is organized into seven chapters covering the anatomical environment of the middle ear, its walls, contents and compartments, the mastoid, the facial nerve, and the Eustachian tube. Subchapters and subdivisions sequentially report and illustrate the related embryology and anatomy, as well as the relevant clinical applications. Basic science is thus directly linked to surgical anatomy and clinical experience, based on the firm view that one must master anatomy in order to adequately perform otological surgery.

The anatomy of the middle ear is explained with numerous color pictures and helpful figures. The book correlates clinical situations to the anatomical basis of diseases and explains the pertinent embryology in order to highlight the buildup of normal anatomy and developmental anomalies. The inclusion of carefully selected CT scans will assist in the reading of normal anatomy and the identification of pathological findings.

This first edition is the result of close collaboration among very good friends who share a strong devotion to medical teaching. It is a tribute to my colleagues' patience and their dedication to selecting the best materials in respect of each topic. I owe them my warmest and most sincere recognition, and many thanks.

Beirut, Lebanon   Prof. Salah Mansour, MD, FRCSC

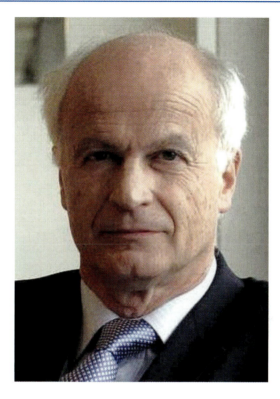

Writing a book is an adventure that can be compared to an expedition in the mountains. You have to gather together material and men, then, instead of hiking, write for a very long time. As the writing goes on, the completion of the book seems all the more distant, just as in climbing the summit seems always farther away. To succeed in such an undertaking, you need a guide, someone who controls the situation and shares his enthusiasm. Salah Mansour has been this unquestioned leader of the expedition. I am but the second in command, there to assure and reassure in case of difficulty.

We met fairly recently, during Salah's visit to Marseille in 1999. His elegance, his culture, and his teaching are captivating. He is surrounded by brilliant students of whom Hassan is one of the most faithful.

One of the main difficulties in mastering otology is not only its complexity but also the diversity of sources that have to be referred to, so as to learn about and understand this specialty thoroughly. Salah and I wasted too much time at the beginning of our career searching for good textbooks, the right information. Hence, our desire is to overcome this obstacle and bring together in one sole reference book the necessary fundamentals to become an otologist.

Thus, this book on the anatomy of the ear, with its detailed descriptions, is completed and illustrated by embryology, pathology, and surgery from our own personal experience. The sole purpose of this book is to fix the boundaries within which the rules of our surgical specialty should evolve. It is up to each practitioner to express himself/herself within these boundaries.

Salah Mansour asked me to participate first in editing the chapter on the external auditory canal, then for the entire book. I thank him for this expression of his trust and friendship.

Marseille, France   Prof. Jacques Magnan, MD, PhD

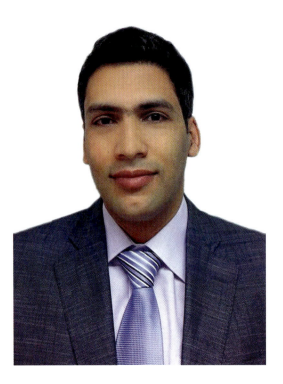

As an otology fellow in training, the junior author, frustrated with available anatomy texts, I was excited to contribute to this work. The encouragement, advises, and recommendations of Professor Mansour and Professor Magnan enabled me to enjoy every demanding step and learn a lot during the writing of a textbook that deals with middle ear embryology, anatomy, radiology, and their clinical relevance. I am convinced that this new book will serve as a sufficient, satisfactory, and complete source to help ambitious otology trainees to overcome many obstacles we faced earlier.

Today this book represents a dream come true. I am grateful for the work of all coauthors who made contributions to this work.

Finally, without the support of my wife, Fatme; my child, Hawraa; and my parents, I would never have succeeded. Although they often had to endure my absence, they seldom complained. I hope they will enjoy the effort being completed.

Marseille, France   Hassan Haidar Ahmad, MD, ABORL

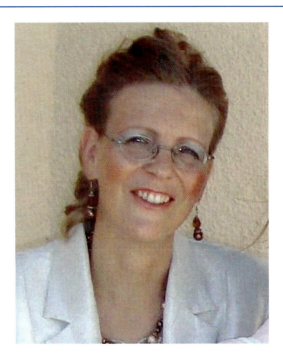

When Professor Mansour invited me to contribute to this book, I was enthusiastic about being associated to this ambitious project.

Nowadays Computed Tomography Scan of the Temporal Bone becomes an accurate and valuable investigation tool for clinical practice, preoperative evaluation, research and teaching in otology.

Having worked for many years in the field of oto-radiology, the great opportunity of clinico-radiological confrontations that I experienced with Professor Mansour and colleagues made me better understand what an otologist is expecting from a CT-Scan in daily practice and in a rich environment of teaching. I succeeded to retain a wide coverage of images enabling me to realize now the objectives of this new book.

CT-Scan offers a precise and excellent identification of the normal anatomic details of the middle ear as well as its pathological conditions, and I hope that this demonstration along the different chapters may encourage any otologist to integrate this diagnostic tool in their daily practice and to benefit from a close correlation between radiological and clinical information.

All my engagements in this field would not have been possible without the generous help of my beloved parents in law, Hanna and Emilie, along with the continuous encouragement and support of my husband and the whole family. I hope that one day my children will experience themselves the passion of combining knowledge and curiosity to get deeper in the secrets of nature.

Beirut, Lebanon   Karen Nicolas, MD

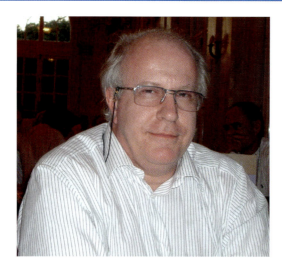

This book is the symbol of a bridge joining distinguished colleagues who shared teaching experience during many years. It results from a close collaboration between various disciplines for the benefit of trainees in the specialty: clinical and basic sciences cooperate to give a comprehensive knowledge of middle ear anatomy in the temporal bone environment. Each structure of the middle ear has its embryological origin. The rules of temporal bone development are very complex but offer a very good understanding of its anatomy. They also permit useful exploration of the relationship with congenital malformations and their interpretation.

The symbol of the bridge corresponds to the necessary and fruitful dialogue between clinicians and fundamental scientists.

This bridge depicts finally the great friendship between the authors.

Brussels, Belgium   Prof. Stéphane Louryan, MD, PhD

Contents

The Temporal Bone

1

Contents

Due to its multiple embryological origins and its adverse developmental aspects, the temporal bone is considered as one of the most complex anatomical structures of the human body. Since the middle ear lodges inside the temporal bone, this chapter will be mostly oriented, not to study the temporal bone as such, but to address it in a specific and restricted scope aiming to describe precisely the developmental and anatomical environment in which the middle ear achieves its final architecture.

The temporal bone houses various cranial nerves and inhabits different important vascular structures and many sensorineural organs in close contacts. Our target will be to demonstrate the richness of such critical structures along with their relationships around and inside the middle ear.

1.1 Embryology of the Temporal Bone

Temporal bone formation results from the fusion and growth of four bones: the squamous, the petrous, the tympanic bones, and the styloid bones. These bones interact to build up the final temporal bone.

Being a part of the skull, temporal bone development is an integral part in the process of skull development. Human skull is developed from three components:

1. *The cartilaginous neurocranium* or *chondrocranium* is the part of the skull formed by endochondral ossification; it constitutes the

S. Mansour et al., *Comprehensive and Clinical Anatomy of the Middle Ear*,
DOI 10.1007/978-3-642-36967-4_1, © Springer-Verlag Berlin Heidelberg 2013

majority of the skull base (ethmoid bone and portions of the occipital, temporal, and sphenoid bones). Endochondral ossification takes place in a cartilaginous anlage; chondroblasts become hypertrophied and progressively change into osteoblasts, which elaborate the bony matrix. The corresponding area is the "ossification center."

2. *The membranous neurocranium or neuroskull* is the part of the skull formed by intramembranous ossification; it constitutes the vault of the skull (frontal, parietal portions of the temporal, occipital, and sphenoid bones). Intramembranous ossification happens when a cluster of mesenchymal cells in a membranous structure gives rise to osteoblasts, in the absence of any cartilaginous matrix.

3. *The viscerocranium or visceroskull* is the part of skull derived from the branchial arches and is suspended to the rest of the cranium [1]. It includes the facial bones.

These three components of the skull contribute actively in the formation of the temporal bone in the following way:

The deep part of the petrous bone is derived from the cartilaginous neurocranium, but the more superficial parts are derived from the membranous neurocranium. The squamous bone is derived from the membranous neurocranium, and the tympanic bone is a part of the visceral skull [2].

1.1.1   Cartilaginous Neurocranium

The majority of the skull base develops from the cartilaginous neurocranium. The formation of the human skull base is a complex process that begins during the fourth week of fetal development. Neural crest cells and paraxial mesoderm derived from occipital somites migrate to sit between the emerging brain and foregut. These cells migrate around and in front of the notochord to form condensations accumulating within the emerging cranial base. The chondrocranium begins to form when these cells condense into cartilage early in the seventh week; these cells are named parachordal cartilages and contribute to the creation of the basal plate.

These parachordal cartilages give rise to the body, greater and lesser wings of the sphenoid bones as well as the perpendicular plate of the ethmoid and the *crista galli*. These embryonic cartilages fuse around the existing cranial nerves and blood vessels to create the primordia of neural foramina [3].

1.1.1.1   The Cartilaginous Otic Capsule

Between the eighth and ninth week of gestation, the cartilaginous otic capsule appears as budge in the base of the cartilaginous cranium. It develops from the mesenchymal tissue that surrounds the otic vesicle. Later the otic capsule becomes surrounded by membranous layers (internal and external periosteal layers); these layers will become the extracapsular part of the petrous bone [3] (Fig. 1.1).

Shortly after this process, the lateral and superior boundaries of the otic capsule begin to appear with the earliest development of the mastoid process and tegmen tympani [4]. A cartilaginous flange grows from the lateral and superior part of the otic capsule and goes downwards and outwards superior to the tubotympanic recess and above the Meckel's cartilage to form the tegmen tympani and the lateral wall of the eustachian tube (ET) (Fig. 1.2) (see Sect. 2.4.1). Thus, the tympanic cavity and the bony part of the ET originate from the petrous bone. Furthermore, from the lateral and inferior part of the cartilaginous otic capsule, another flange grows below the tubotympanic recess to form the jugular plate and the floor of the tympanic cavity. Anteromedially, another periosteal layer grows to form the petrous apex (Fig. 1.2).

By the 16th week, the labyrinth reaches its adult size. Only at this time, the first part of the petrous bone starts to ossify by the endochondral ossification process. There are 14 different ossification centers in the otic capsule, which progressively fuse during the fetal period [4].

The ossification proceeds and continues in the remaining part of the petrous bone to gain its final aspect by about midterm. By the 23rd week of gestation, the rest of the ossification process of the extracapsular parts of the temporal bone continues by extension of the surrounding periosteum forming the mastoid process, the tegmen tympani, middle ear floor, and the walls of the Eustachian

Fig. 1.1 The left temporal bone in a 6 months human fetus. The mastoid area contains external periosteal layer bone (*arrow*), will transform into mastoid bone. Notice that the mastoid antrum (*A*) and the cochlea are already developed. *M* malleus, *I* incus, *EAC* external auditory canal

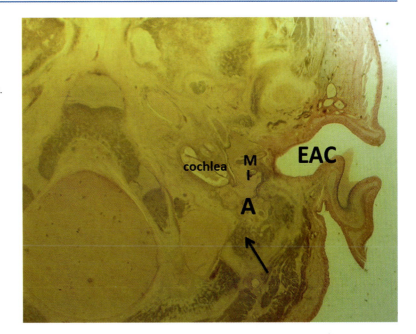

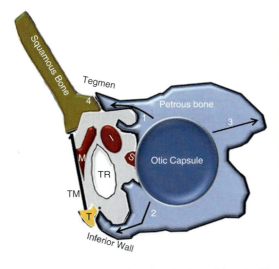

Fig. 1.2 Schematic drawing, frontal plane (34-week-old fetus). Schema showing the cartilaginous flanges running out from the otic capsule: (*1*) lateral and superior flange or the teg-mental plate growing from the otic capsule superior to the tubotympanic recess (*TR*) to form part of the tegmen tympani and the walls of the Eustachian tube; (*2*) lateral and inferior cartilage flange, growing from the otic capsule to form the jugular plate and the floor of the tympanic cavity; (*3*) antero-medial flange growing from the otic capsule anteromedially to form the petrous apex. The inferior wall of the middle ear is built up by the inferior plate of the petrous bone (*2*) which runs laterally to join the tympanic bone (*T*); the plane of fusion con-stitutes the hypotympanic fissure(***). The tympanic bone (*T*) and the tympanic membrane (*TM*) form the lateral wall of the middle ear cavity. The tegmen tympani is formed by fusion of the tegmental process of the petrous bone (*2*) and the transverse plate of the squamous bone (*4*). *M* malleus, *I* incus, *S* stapes

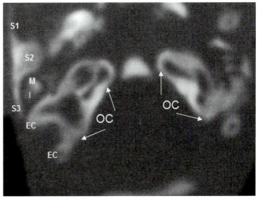

Fig. 1.3 Transversal CT scan of a 22-week-old fetus, show-ing ossification of the otic capsule (*OC*) and beginning of the ossification process in the extracapsular parts of the petrous bone (*EC*) extending to form the mastoid process. The infe-rior part of the squamous bone with its three parts: *S1* anterior part forming the zygomatic process, *S2* middle part forming the roof of the EAC and part of the tegmen, *S3* the posterior part forming the anterior part of the mastoid process. Also notice that the petrous bone and the squamous bone are not yet fused. *M* malleus, *I* incus

tube (Figs. 1.2 and 1.3). The floor of the middle ear ossifies between the 24th and 29th week from an extension of the jugular plate ossification cen-ter [5]. Ossification of the otic capsule is completed only shortly before birth [5].

A delay or a focal lack of the ossification pro-cess may explain the dehiscence of the superior semicircular canal [6, 7].

1.1.2 Membranous Neurocranium and the Squamous Bone

The squamous part of the temporal bone develops from intramembranous ossification; it is formed from one ossification center that appears during the eighth week of gestation [8]. The development of the upper and lower halves of the bone primordium differs:

The upper part is flat and thin and will become the vertical portion.

The lower part, due to the presence of the tympanic bone by the 16th week, bulges and grows rapidly into three directions (Fig. 1.2):

1. *The anterior part* extends anteriorly around the tympanic ring towards the zygomatic bone primordium. It is fixed to the anterosuperior part of the tympanic bone. It forms the zygomatic process of the squamous bone and is involved in the formation of the roof of the temporomandibular joint.
2. *The middle part* sinks medially above the tympanic ring to form the superior wall of the external auditory canal, the attic outer wall, and the lateral part of the tegmen tympani [9].
3. *The posterior part* extends posteriorly behind the tympanic ring to cover a major part of the base of the petrous bone. It forms the anterior portion of the mastoid process.

1.1.3 The Viscerocranium

1.1.3.1 The Styloid Process

The styloid process derives directly from the Reichert's cartilage of the second branchial arch. It develops from two parts:

- The proximal part or the base, also named the tympanohyale, is situated close to the tympanic bone. Its ossification center appears before birth and continues to grow until the age of 4 years. It fuses with the petromastoid component during the first year of life [10].
- The distal part, the stylohyale, starts its ossification only after birth. It fuses with the proximal part only after puberty.

1.1.3.2 The Tympanic Bone

The tympanic ring is a C-shaped bone that provides physical support to the tympanic membrane. It is formed by intramembranous ossification (Fig. 1.4).

At the eighth week of gestation, the tympanic ring appears as a condensation in the cephalic part of the mandibular part of the first branchial arch, which is situated ventral to the first pharyngeal cleft and lateral to Meckel's cartilage. This condensation will extend in a circumferential fashion around the first pharyngeal cleft resulting in the C-shaped structure [11]. Within 2 weeks,

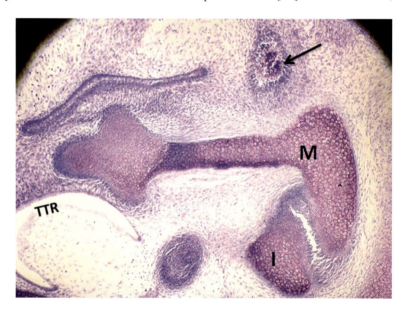

Fig. 1.4 An intramembranous area of ossification (*arrow*) corresponding to the tympanic bone in an E17 mouse embryo (sagittal section, toluidine blue). The cartilaginous primordial of the malleus (*M*) and incus (*I*) are also visible. Tubotympanic recess (*TTR*). Toluidine blue staining at pH4

Fig. 1.5 Skeletal staining of a mouse E 16 embryo. In blue, the Meckel's (*M*) and Reichert's (*R*) cartilages appear in close relationship with the ossicles rudiment (***). In red, we can see maxillary (*Max*) and mandibular (*Man*) bones around the oral cavity (*double arrow*). The tympanic ring (*T*) is also red and ossifies following intramembranous process

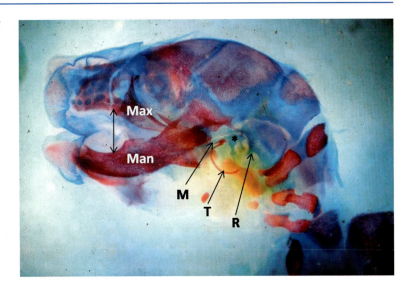

the ossification is first detected in the part of the condensation adjacent to Meckel's cartilage; then it progresses through the rest of the condensation to form a fully developed tympanic ring that is well recognized by the 11th week of gestation (Fig. 1.5).

At 12th week, growth of the tympanic ring proceeds rapidly with a consequent increase in its overall size. The tympanic ring is never closed superiorly, giving rise to the incisura tympanica (*Rivinus notch*) where the pars flaccida of the tympanic membrane will make insertion.

Fusion of the tympanic ring with the other components of the temporal bone starts first at 31st week in the posterior part. The anteromedial segment of the tympanic bone does not join the temporal bone until 37th week. Its fixation to the temporal bone is complete at birth.

The tympanic bone is 9 mm in diameter at birth, almost its definitive size. At this time, it is ring shaped and is open superiorly [12–16].

The formation of the external auditory meatus and the formation of the manubrium are in close association with the tympanic ring formation [11]. The tympanic ring plays an instructive role for the external auditory canal development. Very likely aural atresia results from the failure of the tympanic ring to develop [17]. In addition, the formation of the tympanic ring is essential for the insertion of the manubrium of the

malleus into the tympanic membrane [18]. Several experimental conditions leading to a lack of external auditory meatus formation also result in a severe underdevelopment of the manubrium with a normal aspect of the rest of the malleus. This fact is confirmed in cases of major aural atresia, showing an absence of the manubrium with otherwise normal looking of the rest of the malleus [18, 19].

1.2   Perinatal Changes of the Temporal Bone

By the time the fetus has reached the perinatal period, the squamous and tympanic bones have already fused together; but the resultant segment is still separated from the petrous segment [20]. Early in the perinatal period, these two segments begin to fuse. The fusion of the two segments takes place simultaneously at several locations, beginning with the medial surface of the squamous part to the lateral edge of the tegmental process of the petrous bone. This zone of fusion becomes the internal petrosquamous suture [7]. The fusion continues posteriorly between the petrous and squamous parts of the mastoid process; failure of complete fusion of the two parts leads to formation of a bony septum inside the mastoid process, called Korner's septum [21] (see Sect. 5.1.1). The external petrosquamous suture present on the outer surface of the mastoid process marks the plane of fusion between these two parts.

Finally, the inferior portion of the tympanic ring fuses medially to the inferior process of the petrous bone, thus forming the inferior wall of the tympanic cavity.

1.3   Postnatal Changes of the Temporal Bone

Expansion pressures and antagonist forces exerted by the cephalic neuroskull and the muscular visceroskull, in addition to the pneumatization process, are the main factors for the remodeling process and postnatal changes of the temporal bone.

Bone growth around the tympanic ring following its fusion to the petrous bone proceeds laterally around its circumference. This results in the development of the bony external auditory canal [22]. This lateral extension of the tympanic ring results from the growth of two tympanic tubercles, one from the anterior aspect of the ring and the second from the posterior aspect (Fig. 1.6). These projections grow laterally and then towards each other inferiorly to form the inferior wall of the external auditory canal. By doing so, these projections delimit two openings:

the first is in the upper part, the notch of Rivinus, and the second is inferior, the foramen of Huschke [23].

> **Clinical Pearl**
> Normally the foramen of Huschke closes by the age of 5 years by additional bone growth. This foramen remains patent in about 7 % of adults; in such cases, the skin of the external auditory canal may invaginate into the residual foramen and migrate under the inferior wall of the external bony canal, leading to the formation of a canal cholesteatoma (Fig. 1.7).

Enclosure of the base of the styloid process occurs simultaneously with the lateral extension of the tympanic bone as well.

In addition, the tympanic ring changes its orientation relative to the rest of the cranium.

At birth, the tympanic ring lies beneath the skull in an almost horizontal plane. By the third month, because of the upward and lateral rotation of the petrous bone caused by a rapid enlargement of the forebrain, the tympanic ring appears on the inferolateral aspect of the skull; few months later, it attains its final near vertical orientation [21].

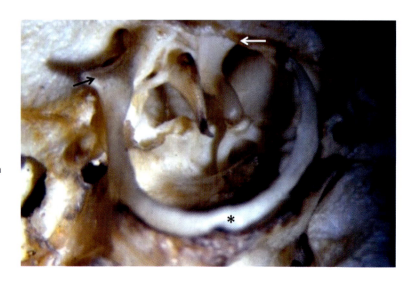

Fig. 1.6 Neonate skull with tympanic annular bone (*) with its anterior tubercle (*white arrow*) and posterior tubercle (*black arrow*). The external auditory meatus is short and ossicles are completely visible

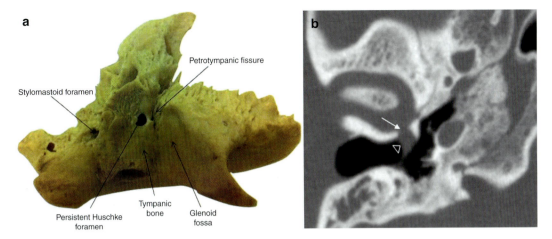

Fig. 1.7 Persistent foramen of Huschke. (**a**) Cadaveric temporal bone, inferior surface, showing a persistent foramen of Huschke. (**b**) Transversal computed tomography of the external auditory canal of a right ear, showing a persistent foramen of Huschke (*white arrow*) with a secondary cholesteatoma (*arrowhead*)

Clinical Pearl

Accompanying the change of orientation of the tympanic bone, changes also occur in tympanic membrane orientation. At birth the tympanic membrane is in almost horizontal plane; this explains the difficulty of exposure of the tympanic membrane in newborns during otoscopic examination or paracentesis. As the tympanic ring changes its orientation, the caudal tympanic sulcus is pushed laterally and the tympanic membrane becomes more vertical.

The styloid process does not make its appearance until after birth. It becomes attached to the tympanic bone during its lateral extension. The progression by which the styloid process grows and ossifies is variable, explaining the variable size and shape of the styloid process in adult skulls [24].

The squamous part of the temporal bone grows rapidly along with the cranial vault during the first 4 years of life and continues at a much slower pace until adulthood [7, 20].

The mastoid process is flat at birth. The stylomastoid foramen is superficial with the facial nerve lying on the lateral surface behind the tympanic bone. Due to pneumatization process in the mastoid process, its lateral portion grows downwards and forwards so that the stylomastoid foramen is pushed medially onto the undersurface of the temporal bone (see Sect. 5.1.2).

1.4   Anatomy of the Temporal Bone

The temporal bone, a paired and symmetrical bone, participates in the formation of the base and of the calvarium of the skull. It is formed from the fusion of four different embryological bones: the petrous bone, the squamous bone, the tympanic bone, and the styloid bone.

The temporal bone is a complex anatomical region that is hollowed by cavities and canals that house the audiovestibular structures and permits the passage of nervous, vascular, and muscular elements. The auditory system is disposed on two axes:

- Anteroposterior air axis consisting of the mastoid antrum, the middle ear cavity, and Eustachian tube
- Latero-medial sensorial axis consisting of the external and internal auditory canals

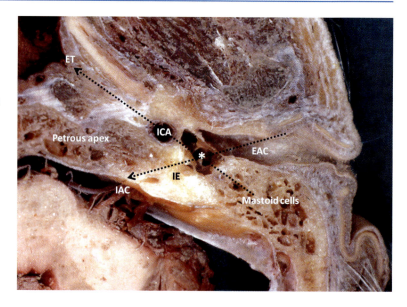

Fig. 1.8 Transverse cut through a left temporal bone showing the middle ear cavity (*) hollowed out in the center of the temporal bone between the external auditory canal (*EAC*) and the inner ear (*IE*). The middle ear lies at the intersection of two axes (*black dotted arrows*), external - internal auditory canal axis and mastoid - Eustachian tube (*ET*) axis. *ICA* internal carotid artery

These two axes intersect at the level of the middle ear cavity (Fig. 1.8).

The temporal bone connects with five other cranial bones: the frontal, parietal, sphenoid, occipital, and zygomatic bone.

1.4.1 The Petrous Bone

Petrous comes from the Latin word "petra" meaning rock; it is the hardest bone of the human skull. It houses the inner ear, the internal carotid artery, the Fallopian canal, and the major part of the middle ear. It results from the ossification of the otic capsule and its flanges.

The petrous bone is shaped like a pyramid that project anteromedially forming a 45° angle with the transverse axis. This pyramid has a posterolateral base (the mastoid) and an anteromedial summit (the petrous apex). It is wedged between the basiocciput and the greater wing of the sphenoid. Its anterosuperior surface is endocranial and participates in the formation of middle cranial fossa floor.

Its posterosuperior surface is also endocranial and forms the anterolateral wall of the posterior cranial fossa. Its inferior surface is exocranial and corresponds to the posteromedial part of the mastoid process.

1.4.2 The Squamous Bone

The squamous bone constitutes the major part of the lateral surface of the temporal bone; it presents a vertical and a horizontal part:

- *The vertical part* is a flat and a thin plate of bone that extends upward to form part of the lateral wall of the middle cranial fossa.
- *The horizontal part* is prolonged anteriorly as the zygomatic process, which originates from two roots: a sagittal posteroexternal root that overhangs the external auditory canal forming its superior part and a transversal anterointernal root that forms the condyle of the temporomandibular joint.

1.4.3 The Tympanic Bone

The tympanic portion of the temporal bone is a gutter-shaped plate of bone. It is situated below the squamous bone between the glenoid fossa anteriorly and the mastoid process posteriorly. The inferior surface of the tympanic bone presents a plate of bone called the vaginal process, which surrounds the styloid process and merges with the petrous bone near the carotid canal.

The tympanic bone forms the anterior, inferior, and posterior walls of the bony external auditory canal. Its attachment to the mastoid and the squamous delineates two suture lines: the tympanosquamous suture anterosuperiorly and the tympanomastoid suture posteroinferiorly. Medially, the tympanic bone articulates with the petrous bone to form the petrotympanic fissure.

The junction between the tympanic bone and the squamous bone superiorly corresponds to the notch of Rivinus.

Medially, the tympanic bone presents a narrow furrow: the tympanic sulcus to which the tympanic membrane annulus is inserted.

1.4.4 The Styloid Bone

The styloid process is a long, slender, and pointed bone of variable length averaging from 20 to 25 mm. It lies anteromedial to the stylomastoid foramen.

The tip of the styloid bone is located between the external and internal carotid arteries, lateral to the pharyngeal wall, and immediately behind the tonsillar fossa.

Three muscles and two ligaments are attached to the styloid process: the stylopharyngeus muscle, the stylohyoid muscle, and the styloglossus muscle. The stylohyoid ligament extends from the tip of the styloid process to the lesser horn of the hyoid bone and the stylomandibular ligament, which starts under the attachment of the styloglossus muscle and ends on the mandibular angle [10, 22, 25–27].

> **Clinical Pearl**
> The ossification process of the styloid ligament may involve the whole length of the ligament, giving rise to a bony prolongation between the skull and the hyoid bone; this may manifest clinically by odynophagia, Eagle's syndrome (Fig. 1.9).

1.4.5 Temporal Bone Fissures

Four intrinsic fissures form at the fusion lines of the four bones forming the temporal bone.

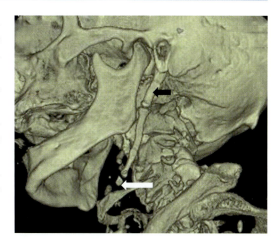

Fig. 1.9 Computed tomography with 3D reformation showing complete ossification of the stylohyoid ligament from the styloid process (*upper arrow*) to its insertion on the hyoid bone (*lower arrow*)

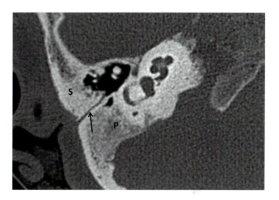

Fig. 1.10 Transversal computed tomography of the right temporal bone of a child with hereditary cleidocranial dysostosis: prominent petrosquamous suture (*black arrow*) that could be misinterpreted as a temporal bone fracture. *S* squamous bone, *P* petrous bone

1.4.5.1 The Petrosquamous Fissure

The petrosquamous fissure or suture connects the petrous bone and the squamous bone and opens directly into the mastoid antrum. It is a narrow fissure and continuous with the petrotympanic fissure.

The external petrosquamous fissure, which links the squamous and the petrous parts of the mastoid process, is sometimes visible on the outer surface of the mastoid process (Fig. 1.10). The internal petrosquamous fissure is located in the tegmen tympani and joins its squamous and petrous portions.

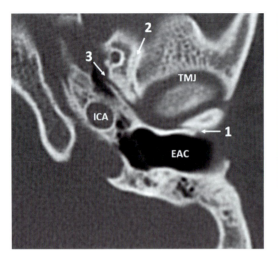

Fig. 1.11 Transversal computed tomography of a left ear, showing the three different sutures appearing with an Y shape. They form together the Glaserian fissure. *1* the tympanosquamous fissure, *2* the anterior petrosquamous fissure, *3* the petrotympanic fissure. *ICA* internal carotid artery, *EAC* external auditory canal, *TMJ* temporomandibular joint

1.4.5.2 Tympanomastoid Fissure

The tympanomastoid fissure or suture anchors the tympanic bone to the mastoid process.

This suture is situated in the posteroinferior part of the external auditory canal (see Fig. 1.12).

The auricular branch of the vagus nerve, Arnold nerve, emerges through the tympanomastoid suture to innervate part of the external auditory canal skin.

1.4.5.3 Tympanosquamous Fissure

The tympanosquamous fissure connects the tympanic bone to the squamous bone.

The tympanosquamous fissure is seen in the anterosuperior part of the external auditory canal and continues medially into the petrotympanic and petrosquamous fissures (see Figs. 1.11 and 1.12).

1.4.5.4 The Petrotympanic Fissure

The petrotympanic fissure or Glaserian fissure is situated between the medial aspect of the tympanic bone and the mandibular fossa. It transmits the chorda tympani, the anterior tympanic artery, and the anterior malleal ligament (Fig. 1.11).

Clinical Pearl

In the context of trauma, these normal fissures, especially if evident, may be misinterpreted as temporal bone fractures (Figs. 1.10 and 1.11).

The petrosquamous fissure may remain open until the age of 20 years, providing a route for a spread of infection from the middle ear to the intracranial cavity.

1.4.6 Temporal Bone Surfaces

The temporal bone exhibits four surfaces: the lateral, posterior, superior, and inferior surface.

1.4.6.1 The Lateral Surface (Fig. 1.12)

The squama constitutes the major part of the lateral surface of the temporal bone and extends upward as a flat bone to cover part of the temporal lobe of the cerebrum.

The lateral surface of the squama shows a vertical groove for the middle temporal artery and serves as an area of attachment for the temporalis muscle.

The medial surface of squama is grooved for the branches of the middle meningeal artery. Inferior to the squama, the external auditory canal is located. The tympanic bone forms the anterior, inferior, and posterior walls of the bony external auditory canal. The hiatus between the tympanic bone and the squamous bone corresponds to the *notch of Rivinus*. Anterior to the external auditory canal is the temporomandibular joint; a thin bony shell separates them from each other.

Several important landmarks mark the lateral surface of the temporal bone:

- *The mastoid process* refers to the bony process located on the posteroinferior border of the lateral surface of the temporal bone. Two distinct bones contribute to the formation of the mastoid process: the anterosuperior portion is formed by squamous bone and the petrous bone forms the posteroinferior portion. These processes serve laterally for the attachment of the sternocleidomastoid muscle and medially to the posterior belly of the digastric muscle (see Sect. 5.2).

Fig. 1.12 Lateral surface of a left temporal bone. *1* tympanosquamous fissure, *2* tympanomastoid fissure, *EAC* external auditory canal, *S* Henle's spine, * suprameatal triangle, *VP* vaginal process

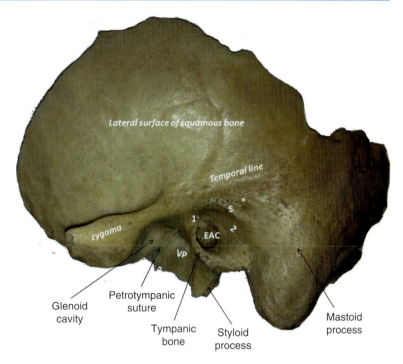

• *The zygomatic process* originates above the external auditory canal. It leaves the squama and projects anteriorly to unite the zygomatic bone. On the inferior surface of the zygomatic process is the mandibular or glenoid fossa, which accommodates the condyle of the mandible. The anterior limit of the glenoid fossa is demarcated by the articular eminence; the post-glenoid process demarcates its posterior limit. The glenoid fossa communicates with the middle ear through the petrotympanic fissure.

• *The temporal line or supramastoid crest*: posterior to the external auditory canal the zygomatic process prolongs as a faint line or the supramastoid crest. This crest serves for the attachment of the temporal muscle. It is an important landmark for the level of middle cranial fossa dura.

• *Suprameatal Mac-Ewen's triangle*: located between the posterosuperior wall of the external auditory canal and the temporal line. This triangle corresponds medially to the antrum.

• *Henle's spine*: it is a bony spine implanted on the posterosuperior edge of the external auditory canal; it corresponds to the attic medially.

• *The scutum* is a sharp bony spur formed at the junction of the lateral wall of the middle ear cavity and the superior wall of the external auditory canal which is part of the squamous bone.

1.4.6.2 Posterior Surface

The posterior surface of the temporal bone is formed exclusively by the petrous part. It represents the anterolateral wall of the posterior cranial fossa. This surface is limited superiorly by the sulcus for the superior petrosal venous sinus, which separates the superior and the posterior surfaces of the petrous bone. Laterally it presents the sigmoid sinus sulcus and the internal orifice of the emissary vein canal.

The most important feature of the posterior surface is the internal auditory meatus, which lies in the center of this surface midway between the apex and the anterior border of the sigmoid sinus sulcus. An important structure situated at the lateral part of this surface is the endolymphatic sac; this sac lies medial to

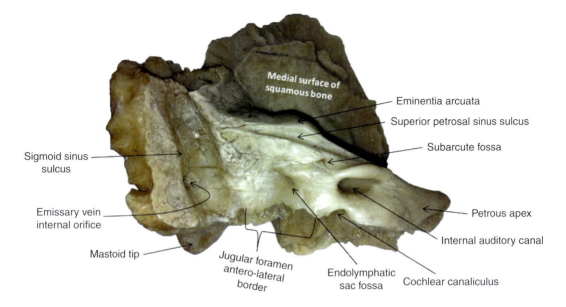

Fig. 1.13 Posterior surface of a left temporal bone

Fig. 1.14 Posterior surface of a right temporal bone showing the relation of the internal auditory canal (*) with the sigmoid sinus (*black arrow*), the middle cranial fossa (*MCF*) (*white arrow*), and the jugular bulb (*JB*). *SPS* superior petrosal sinus, *IPS* inferior petrosal sinus, *PA* petrous apex, *V* fifth CN, *VI* sixth cranial nerve in Dorello's canal, *IX, X, XI* ninth, tenth, and eleventh CN

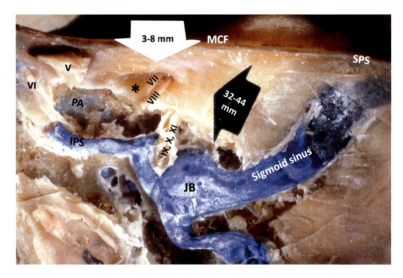

the level of the posterior semicircular canal (Fig. 1.13).

The average dimensions of the internal auditory canal are 1 cm horizontally and 0.5 cm vertically. The mean distance from the highest border of the jugular bulb to the inferior border of the internal auditory canal is about 0.5 cm [28] (Fig. 1.14). The mean distance from the lateral border of the internal auditory canal to the endolymphatic sac is about 1 cm [29].

Surgical Implications

During retrosigmoid approach for hearing preservation surgery in vestibular schwannoma, drilling of the posterior lip of the internal auditory canal may be necessary in order to remove the intrameatal portion of the tumor. This step carries a risk of injuring the posterior semicircular canal or a high riding jugular bulb.

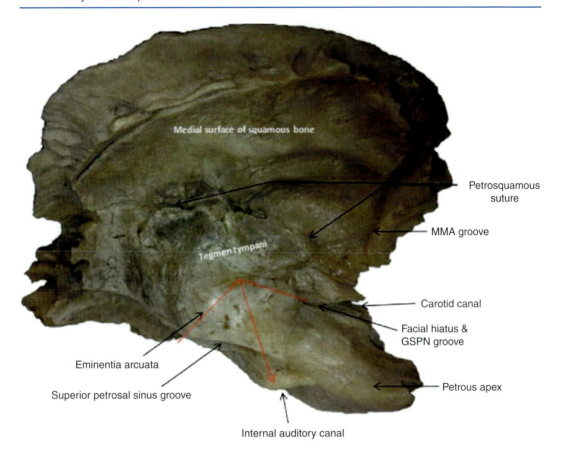

Medial surface of squamous bone

Petrosquamous suture

MMA groove

Tegmen tympani

Carotid canal

Facial hiatus & GSPN groove

Eminentia arcuata

Superior petrosal sinus groove

Petrous apex

Internal auditory canal

Fig. 1.15 Superior view of a left temporal bone. The red lines represent the relation of the internal auditory canal with respect to the eminencia arcuata and the greater superficial petrosal nerve (*GSPN*), middle meningeal artery (*MMA*)

Based on these measurements mentioned above, 0.5 cm of bone can be safely drilled away from the posterior lip of the canal without injuring any structure.

1.4.6.3 Superior Surface (Fig. 1.15)

The superior surface of the temporal bone forms part of the middle cranial fossa floor; it is limited posteromedially by the superior petrosal sinus sulcus.

The superior surface presents from lateral to medial several structures that serve as important surgical landmarks during middle cranial fossa approach.

Tegmen Tympani

The most lateral part of this surface contains the tegmen tympani, which separates the middle cranial fossa from the middle ear. It is formed partly from the caudal portion of the squamous bone, which extends medially to join the petrous bone. The petrous bone forms the major part of the tegmen. The fusion line of the two bones forms the petrosquamous fissure.

Eminentia Arcuata

The Eminentia arcuata is an important surgical landmark. It lies on the posterior part of the superior surface, near the superior petrosal sinus, about 20–25 mm from the inner tablet of the cranium [30, 31]. It corresponds to the wall of the superior semicircular canal. Usually the posterior aspect of the eminentia arcuata is rotated lateral to the posterior crus of the superior semicircular canal, but the anterior aspect of the eminentia arcuata is located over the anterior crus of this canal [30, 32].

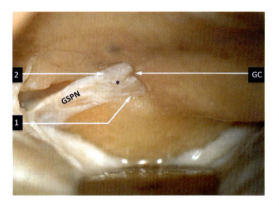

Fig. 1.16 Middle cranial fossa view of a right-side facial nerve. View after drilling off the bone covering the geniculate ganglion (*). G.C., geniculate crest; (*1*) labyrinthine segment of facial nerve; (*2*) tympanic segment of facial nerve (Courtesy of Tardivet [36])

Greater Superficial Petrosal Nerve and Geniculate Ganglion (Fig. 1.16)

The superior surface is marked also by the facial hiatus and the groove of the greater superficial petrosal nerve, which runs from the geniculate ganglion to the middle cranial fossa. The distance from the geniculate ganglion and the inner tablet of the cranium is of 2.7 mm. Two plates of bone form the bony roof of the geniculate ganglion and the proximal part of the greater superficial petrosal nerve bony canal: a medial plate, which is a periosteal derivative of the petrous bone, and a lateral plate, which is a membranous derivative from the squamous bone.

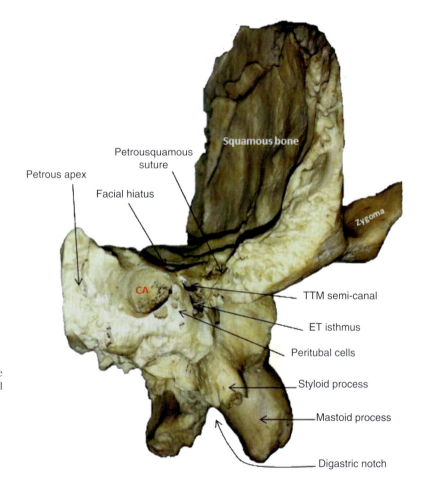

Fig. 1.17 Anteromedial view of a left petrous bone showing the petrous apex and the exit orifice of the carotid canal (*CA*) from the temporal bone anterolateral to the petrous apex. Notice the position of the ET isthmus and the tensor tympani muscle (*TTM*) semicanal lateral to the carotid canal

The geniculate ganglion could be dehiscent in 15–20 % of cases. In these cases, the risk of injuring the facial nerve during middle cranial fossa approach is very high while elevating of the dura mater from the superior surface of the temporal bone [30, 33, 34].

In middle cranial fossa approach, the internal auditory meatus is within 3–8 mm distant from the superior border of the petrous bone. The bisection of the angle formed by the greater superior petrosal nerve and the eminence arcuate marks the position of the internal auditory meatus (Fig. 1.14).

The Petrous Apex

The petrous apex is situated in the angular interval between the posterior border of the sphenoid and the basilar part of the occipital bone. The main portion of the apex lies anterior to the cochlea. Through the *apex*, the internal carotid artery exits the petrous bone to the foramen lacerum, which is found between the apex and the sphenoid bone (Fig. 1.17).

1.4.6.4 Inferior Surface (Fig. 1.18)

The inferior surface of the temporal bone represents posterolaterally the inferior part of the mastoid and the digastric notch. Anterior to the digastric notch and posterior to the styloid process is the stylomastoid foramen, from which the facial nerve leaves the temporal bone. Medial to the digastric notch is a shallow groove for the occipital artery.

More anteriorly lies the inferior surface of the tympanic bone, which forms the posterior boundary of the mandibular fossa and expands inferiorly to form the vaginal process.

Anteromedial to the stylomastoid foramen and styloid process is the jugular foramen; it is formed by the petrous bone anterolaterally and the occipital bone posteromedially.

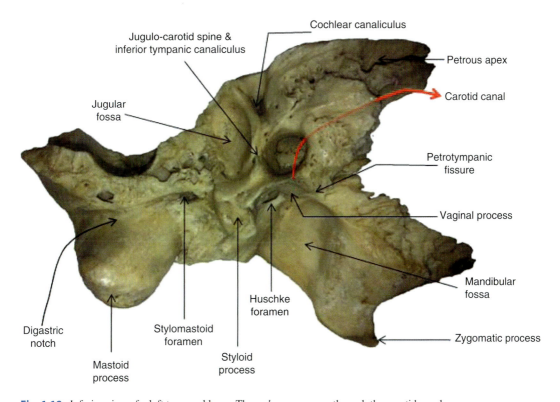

Fig. 1.18 Inferior view of a left temporal bone. The *red arrow* passes through the carotid canal

The jugular foramen is separated by the jugular spine and a fibrous band into two fibro-osseous compartments:

- Pars vascularis: posterolateral vascular compartment, which is larger and receives the internal jugular vein, vagus nerve (CN X) with Arnold's branch, the spinal nerve (CN XI), and posterior meningeal artery
- Pars nervosa: anteromedial nervous compartment, which is smaller and receives the glossopharyngeal nerve (CN IX) with its Jacobson's branch and the inferior petrosal sinus [35]

Posterior to the jugular fossa lies the small canal of Arnold's nerve.

Medial to the jugular fossa, there is the groove of the inferior petrosal sinus and the opening of the cochlear aqueduct.

The foramen of the internal carotid artery lies anterior to the jugular foramen and is separated from its anterior border by the jugulo-carotid spine through which we find a canal for the passage of Jacobson's nerve (IX) to the tympanic cavity.

Medially, near the petrous apex, the inferior surface presents the site of insertion of the levator veli palatini and the cartilaginous portion of the Eustachian tube.

References

1. Leland Albright A, David Adelson P, Pollack F. Principles and practice of pediatric neurosurgery, vol. 2. New York: Thieme Publishers; 2007. p. 668–9.
2. Le Douarin NM, Kalcheim C. The neural crest. 2nd ed. Cambridge: Cambridge University Press; 1999.
3. Doden E, Halves R. On the functional morphology of the human petrous bone. Am J Anat. 1984;169(4): 451–62.
4. Bast TH. Ossification of the optic capsule in human fetuses. Washington, D.C.: Carnegie Institution of Washington; 1930.
5. Dahm MC, Shepherd RK, Clark GM. The postnatal growth of the temporal bone and its implications for cochlear implantation in children. Acta Otolaryngol Suppl. 1993;505:1–39.
6. Zhou G, Ohlms I, Ohlms I, Amin M. Superior semicircular canal dehiscence in a young child; implication of development defect. Int J Pediatr Otorhinolaryngol. 2007;71(12):1925–8.
7. Jacquot S, Bertholon P, Chaudron S, Prade J-M, Martin C. Dehiscence du canal semi-circulaire supérieur. Fr ORL. 2006;91:249–25610.
8. Tortori-Donati P, Rossi A, editors. Pediatric neuroradiology: brain, head, neck, and spine. New York: Springer; 2005. p. 1255–65.
9. Schuknecht H. Pathology of the ear. Cambridge: Harvard University Press; 1974. p. 503.
10. Monsour PA, Young WG. Variability of the styloid process and stylohyoid ligament in panoramic radiographs. Oral Med Oral Pathol. 1986;61:522–6.
11. Mallo M, Gridley T. Development of the mammalian ear: coordinate regulation of formation of the tympanic ring and the external acoustic meatus. Development. 1996;122:173–9.
12. Ars B, Decraemer W, Marquet J, Ars-Piret N. Sulcustympanicus. In: Comptes-rendusduCongrès de la Société Française d'ORL. Paris: Arnette; 1980. p. 401–68.
13. Ars B, Ars-Piret N. Mouvements embryogéniques de l'anneau tympanique. In: Martin H, editor. Comptes rendus du Congrès de la Société Française d'ORL. Paris: Arnette; 1981. p. 117–9.
14. Ars B. Pars TympanicaOssisTemporalis. Academical-thesis, thèse d'agrégation de l'Enseignement supérieur. University of Antwerp; 1982.
15. Ars B. La partie tympanale de l'os temporal. Cahiers ORL. 1983;18:435–523.
16. Anson BJ, Bast TH, Richamy SF. The fetal and early postnatal development of the tympanic ring and related structures in man. Ann Otol Rhinol Laryngol. 1955;64:802–22.
17. Michaels L, Soucek S. Development of the stratified squamous epithelium of the human tympanic membrane and external canal: the origin of auditory epithelial migration. Am J Anat. 1989;184:334–44.
18. Mallo M, Schrewe H, Martin JF, Olson EN, Ohnemus S. Assembling a functional tympanic membrane: signals from the external acoustic meatus coordinate development of the malleal manubrium. Development. 2000;127(19):4127–36.
19. Yamada G, Mansouri A, Torres M, Stuart ET, Blum M, Schultz M, De Robertis EM, Gruss P. Targeted mutation of the murine goosecoid gene results in craniofacial defects and neonatal death. Development. 1995;121(9):2917–22.
20. Eby TL, Nadol JB. Postnatal growth of the human temporal bone. Implications for cochlear implants in children. Ann Otol Rhinol Laryngol. 1986;95: 356–64.
21. Wright A. Anatomy and ultrastructure of the human ear, chapter 1. In: Kerr GA, editor. Scott Brown's otolaryngology, vol. 1. 6th ed. London: Butterworth Heinemann; 1997. p. 1–50.
22. Gulya AJ. Developmental anatomy of the temporal bone and skull base. In: Glasscock ME, Gulya AJ, editors. Glasscock-Shambaugh Surgery of the Ear. 5th ed. Hamilton: BC Decker Inc; 2003. p. 4–7.
23. Ars B. Foramen of huschke. Valsalva. 1984;60(3): 205–11.

24. Simms DL, Neely JG. Growth of the lateral surface of the temporal bone in children. Laryngoscope. 1989;99(8 Pt 1):795–9.

25. Moffat DA, Ramsden RT, Shaw HJ. The styloid process syndrome: aetiological factors and surgical management. J Laryngol Otol. 1977; 91(4):279–94.

26. Jung T, Tschernitschek H, Hippen H, Schneider B, Borchers L. Elongated styloid process: when is it really elongated? Dentomaxillofac Radiol. 2004;33(2): 119–24.

27. Gözil R, Yener N, Calgüner E, Araç M, Tunç E, Bahcelioğlu M. Morphological characteristics of styloid process evaluated by computerized axial tomography. Ann Anat. 2001;183(6):527–35.

28. Kolagi S, Herur A, Ugale M, Manjula R, Mutalik A. Suboccipital retrosigmoid surgical approach for internal auditory canal–a morphometric anatomical study on dry human temporal bones. Indian J Otolaryngol Head Neck Surg. 2010;62(4):372–5.

29. Koval J, Molcan M, Bowdler AD, Sterkers JM. Retrosigmoid transmeatal approach: an anatomic study of an approach used for preservation of hearing in acoustic neuroma surgery and vestibular neurotomy. Skull Base Surg. 1993;3(1):16–21.

30. Chopra R, Fergie N, Mehta D, Liew L. The middle cranial fossa approach: an anatomical study. Surg Radiol Anat. 2003;24(6):348–51; discussion 352–3.

31. Clerc P, Batisse R. [Approach to the intrapetrosal organs by the endocranial route; graft of the facial nerve]. Ann Otolaryngol. 1954;71(1):20–38.

32. Kartush JM, Kemink JL, Graham MD. The arcuate eminence. Topographic orientation in middle cranial fossa surgery. Ann Otol Rhinol Laryngol. 1985;94 (1 Pt 1):25–8.

33. Dobozi M. Surgical anatomy of the Geniculate ganglion. Acta Otolaryngol. 1975;80(1–2):116–9.

34. Rhoton Jr AL, Pulec JL, Hall GM, Boyd Jr AS. Absence of bone over the geniculate ganglion. J Neurosurg. 1968;28(1):48–53.

35. Roche PH, Mercier P, Sameshima T, Fournier HD. Surgical anatomy of the jugular foramen. Adv Tech Stand Neurosurg. 2008;33:233–63.

36. Tardivet L. Anatomie Chirurgicale du nerf facial intra-petreux, Thèse Med. Aix Marseille University; 2003.

Middle Ear Cavity

2

Contents

The middle ear cavity is an irregular air-filled space hollowed out in the center of the temporal bone between the external auditory meatus laterally and the inner ear medially (Fig. 2.1). It lies at the intersection between two important axes: one latero-medial between the external and the internal auditory canals, the other one posteroanterior between the mastoid antrum and the Eustachian tube (see Fig. 1.8).

For descriptive purposes, the tympanic cavity may be considered as a box with four walls, a roof, and a floor. Because of the convexity of the medial and lateral walls, the middle ear cavity is constricted at its center. The width of the middle ear cavity is 2 mm at the center, 6 mm superiorly in the attic, and 4 mm inferiorly in the hypotympanum. In the sagittal plane, the middle ear cleft measures about 15 mm both in the vertical and horizontal directions (Fig. 2.2).

The middle ear cavity is surrounded by six walls: the lateral wall, the inferior wall called the floor or the jugular wall, the posterior called the mastoid wall, the superior wall also called the roof or the tegmen, the anterior wall called the carotid wall, and the medial wall called the cochlear wall.

2.1 Lateral Wall

The lateral wall is formed by the tympanic membrane, the bony tympanic ring and the attic outer wall (Fig. 2.2). This wall of the middle ear cavity,

Fig. 2.1 Oblique cut of a right temporal bone. The middle ear cavity lies in the center of the temporal bone between the outer ear (*EAC*) and the inner ear. *T* the tympanic membrane, *i* incus; *m* malleus, *sscc* superior semicircular canal, *ET* Eustachian tube, *IAC* internal auditory canal, *ICA* internal carotid artery

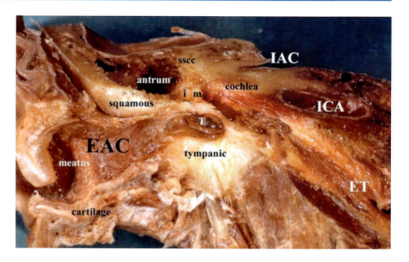

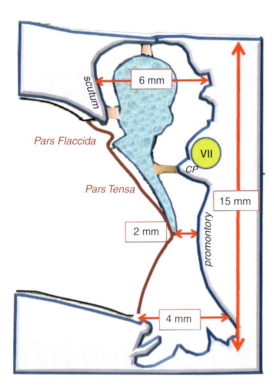

Fig. 2.2 Schematic drawing of the middle ear cavity showing its different dimensions. *VII* facial nerve, *CP* cochleariform process

especially the tympanic membrane, is the only wall accessible to clinical examination and is the site of most middle ear pathologies. In addition, the lateral wall represents the classic entry site to the middle ear during ear surgery.

2.1.1   Embryology of the Lateral Wall

The development of the tympanic bone and membrane starts as early as the fourth week of intrauterine life [1]. A funnel-shaped ectoblastic pouch grows inwards from the first branchial cleft until it reaches an endoblastic pouch growing laterally from the first branchial pouch, known as the tubotympanic recess. The contact between the ectoblastic and the endoblastic pouches is short-living.

By the fifth week of the fetal life and due to the growth of the cephalic extremity with its flexion-extension positions, the region of the future neck creates two types of forces: an expansive force and a depressive force. Under the expansive cephalic flexion, the mesenchyme interposes between the ectoblastic and the endoblastic pouches. At the seventh week this mesenchyme contributes to the formation of the fibrous stratum of the tympanic membrane and the handle of malleus (Fig. 2.3).

At the eighth week, the epithelial cells at the bottom of the ectoblastic pouch proliferate and form a compact epithelial plate reaching the endoblast. Later, this ectoblastic plate gives rise to the bony external auditory canal and the tympanic membrane at its end. When the tympanic membrane appears, it consists already of three layers and has an elliptical form with a horizontal diameter of approximately 2 mm.

At birth the tympanic membrane is in almost horizontal plane. As the tympanic ring changes its

Fig. 2.3 Tympanic membrane formation. The tympanic membrane is formed from the three germ layers, ectoderm (*1*), mesoderm (*2*), and endoderm (*3*)

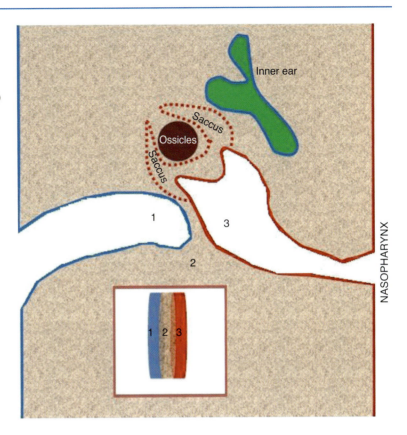

orientation, the caudal tympanic sulcus is pushed laterally and the tympanic membrane becomes more vertical (see Sect. 1.3). This explains the difficulty of exposure of the tympanic membrane in newborns during otoscopic examination or paracentesis.

Clinical Pearl

Congenital Cholesteatoma

Congenital cholesteatoma are residual squamous inclusion cysts that arise from epithelial rests in the middle ear. These epithelial rests are normally seen during fetal development and usually disappear by the third trimester. The failed involution of these epithelial rests leads to a congenital cholesteatoma [2, 3].

2.1.2   Lateral Wall Anatomy

The lateral wall of the tympanic cavity is partly bony and partly membranous. The central portion of the lateral wall is formed by the tympanic membrane and the incomplete tympanic ring to which the membrane is attached. Above the tympanic membrane there is a bony wall forming the attic outer wall.

2.1.2.1   The Attic Outer Wall

The attic outer wall, part of the squamous bone, is the bony lateral wall of the attic. It is a wedge-shaped plate of bone that separates the attic from the zygomatic mastoid cells laterally (Fig. 2.4).

The part of the attic outer wall lying below the plane tracing the roof of the external auditory canal is called the *scutum* (means shield in Latin).

The scutum is a thin sharp bony spur formed by the junction of the attic outer wall and the superior wall of the external auditory canal. The scutum forms part of the superior deep portion of the external meatus and gives attachment to the pars flaccida of the tympanic membrane, which is the lateral wall of the Prussak's space (Fig. 2.4).

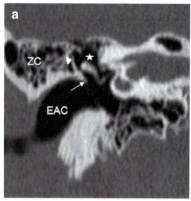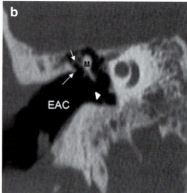

Fig. 2.4 (**a**) Coronal reconstruction of a computed tomography of a right ear, showing the scutum as a sharp bony spur (*white arrow*) and the attic outer wall (*white arrowhead*) that separates the attic (*) from the zygomatic cells (*ZC*). (**b**) Coronal computed tomography reconstruction of a right ear: erosion of the scutum (*long arrow*), due to a retraction pocket in the Prussak's space with keratin debris (*short arrow*). Thickened tympanic membrane (*arrowhead*); *M* malleus, *EAC* external auditory canal

---

Clinical Impact
The scutum is the first bony structure to be eroded by an attical cholesteatoma secondary to a retraction pocket of the pars flaccida into the attic (Fig. 2.4b).

2.1.2.2 The Tympanic Ring

The tympanic ring is the most medial portion of the tympanic bone; it is C shaped and represents the frame in which inserts most of the tympanic membrane periphery. In the inner aspect of the tympanic ring, there is a gutter, the *tympanic sulcus*, which houses the *annulus* of the tympanic membrane.

The tympanic ring is deficient superiorly to form the *notch of Rivinus*. The pars flaccida inserts directly on this notch, and due to the absence of sulcus and the tympanic ring, the pars flaccida is lax rendering it more predisposed to a retraction (Fig. 2.5).

The Tympanic Spines

At the junction of the tympanic ring and the attic outer wall, we can identify two spines – the anterior and the posterior tympanic spines (Fig. 2.5):
1. *Anterior tympanic spine:* is present at the anterosuperior end of the tympanic ring and represents the anterior limit of the notch of Rivinus
2. *Posterior tympanic spine:* is present at the posterosuperior end of the tympanic ring and represents the posterior limit of the notch of Rivinus

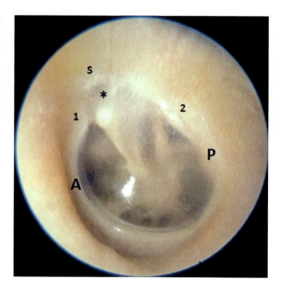

Fig. 2.5 Left tympanic membrane showing the notch of Rivinus (*) limited by the anterior (*1*) and posterior (*2*) tympanic spines. Notice the direct insertion of the tympanic membrane on the scutum (*s*) and the absence of annulus in this zone. Also notice the difference in size between the anterior part of the annulus (*A*) and the posterior part (*P*) of the annulus

Tympanic Canaliculi

The medial surface of the tympanic ring near the tympanic spines presents three openings (Fig. 2.6):
- *The Petrotympanic Fissure (Glaserian Fissure)*
  The petrotympanic (Glaserian) fissure opens anteriorly just above the attachment of the

Fig. 2.6 Schematic drawing of the medial surface of a right tympanic membrane showing Glaserian fissure containing the anterior malleal ligament (*AML*), the more medial canal of Huguier giving exit for the chorda tympani to the infratemporal fossa. The chorda tympani enters the middle ear through the iter chordæ posterius

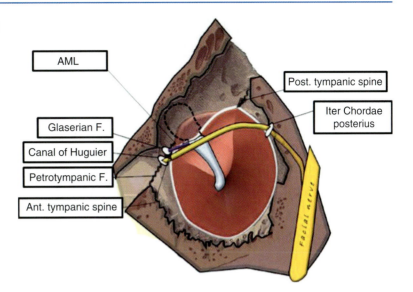

tympanic membrane. It is a slit about 2 mm long, which receives the anterior malleal ligament and transmits the anterior tympanic artery, a branch of the internal maxillary artery to the tympanic cavity (see Fig. 1.11).

- *The Iter Chordæ Anterius* (*Canal of Huguier*)
  The canal of Huguier is a separate canaliculus placed in the medial end of the petrotympanic fissure; through it the chorda tympani nerve leaves the tympanic cavity towards the infratemporal fossa.
- *The Iter Chordæ Posterius*
  The iter chordæ posterius is situated medial to the posterior tympanic spine. It leads into a minute canal through which the chorda tympani nerve exits to enter the tympanic cavity. It lies immediately medial to the tympanic membrane at the level of the upper limit of the malleus handle.

The Tympanic Sulcus

The tympanic sulcus houses the annulus of the tympanic membrane. The lateral edge of the tympanic sulcus is higher than the medial edge.

The average depth of the sulcus is about 1 mm. However, this depth is not constant; it is maximal at 6 o'clock and decreases gradually as it goes up towards the tympanic spines where it disappears completely. The posterosuperior part of the sulcus is shallow and its depth is around 4 mm.

Clinical Implications

These changes in the depth of the sulcus reflect the stability of the insertion of the annulus; in the posterosuperior quadrant the annulus is not totally inserted into the sulcus and is merely supported (Fig. 2.7). This weak insertion of the posterosuperior quadrant of tympanic membrane to the tympanic ring makes it lax and predisposed to retraction [4].

2.1.2.3 The Tympanic Membrane

The tympanic membrane (TM) separates the external auditory meatus from the middle ear. It is a thin semitransparent membrane that is nearly circular in form and is approximately 8 mm wide, 9–10 mm high, and 0.1 mm thick.

The inferior part of the membrane lies more medially than the superior part; the TM forms an inclination of about 40° relative to the inferior wall of the auditory meatus (Figs. 2.1 and 2.8).

The handle of the malleus is firmly attached to the central part of the inner surface of the TM and draws it centrally; this zone of the TM is called the *umbo* (Fig. 2.10).

Shrapnell divided the TM into two parts, an upper small part called *pars flaccida* and a lower bigger part called the *pars tensa*.

Fig. 2.7 A medial view of the lateral wall of a left middle ear showing the incomplete insertion of the posterosuperior part of the annulus (*white arrow*) in the tympanic sulcus. *1* iter chordæ posterius, *2* iter chordæ anterius, *FI* fossa incudis, *TM* tympanic membrane, *M* malleus, *I* incus, * chorda tympani

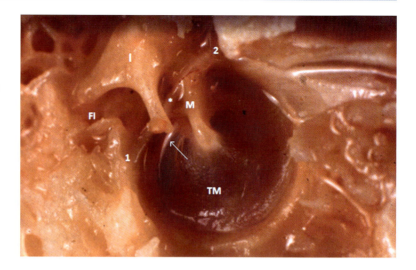

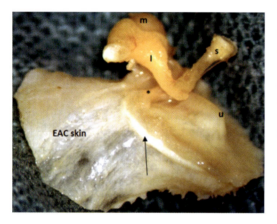

Fig. 2.8 Left ear tympanic membrane allograft showing the annulus (*black arrow*) and the posterior tympano-malleal fold (*). *I* incus, *m* malleus, *u* umbo, *s* stapes

The *pars tensa*, the largest part of the TM, is taut, thickened peripherally into the annulus which is inserted into the tympanic sulcus.

The *pars flaccida*, Shrapnell's membrane, is lax, occupies the notch of Rivinus, and is attached to the scutum [5].

The Tympanic Annulus

The tympanic annulus, or Gerlach's ligament is a horseshoe-like fibrocartilaginous structure that maintains the insertion of the tympanic membrane in the tympanic sulcus (Fig. 2.8). The annulus is absent superiorly at the level of the notch of Rivinus.

In cross section, the annulus shows a triangular form with a summit pointing towards the pars tensa and a base inserted on the tympanic sulcus [6].

At the level of the tympanic spines, the tympanic annulus prolongs centrally towards the lateral process of the malleus constituting two strands: the anterior and the posterior tympano-malleal strands. These two strands divide the tympanic membrane into the pars flaccida superiorly and the pars tensa inferiorly. Medially, these two strands rise up two slight ridges of mucous membrane on the inner side of the tympanic membrane called the *anterior* and *posterior tympano-malleolar folds* (Fig. 2.8).

The diameter of the annulus is not uniform. The maximal mean caliber of the annulus is at 6 o'clock level; from this point, the annulus gradually thins out in both directions until it reaches about 15 % of its maximal caliber at the anterior and posterior tympanic spines [4, 7] (Fig. 2.5).

Surgical Application

During middle ear surgery, the annulus allows an operative dislocation of the tympanic membrane out of the sulcus without tearing it. The most difficult part of the annulus to dislodge is the anterior part because of its firm attachment to the sulcus.

Microscopic Structure
of the Tympanic Membrane

The pars tensa and pars flaccida differ in structure despite the fact that both parts are made of three layers: a lateral epidermal layer, a medial mucosal layer, and a middle layer or lamina propria.

- *The epidermal layer*
  The epidermis of the TM and of the bony part of the external ear canal is a specialized type of skin; it does not contain any glands or hair follicles, and it has a potential of lateral migration not encountered in any epidermis elsewhere. Epithelial cells migrate centrifugally outwards from the center of the drum desquamating only when they reach the cartilaginous portion of the ear canal. This process accounts for the self-cleaning ability of the ear canal [8].

- *The Mucosal layer*
  The mucosal layer of the eardrum is a continuation of the mucosal lining of the middle ear cavity. It is a very thin monocellular layer of cells.

- *Lamina propria*
  This intermediate layer consists of fibrous tissue: The amount and the organization of this tissue is the main difference between the pars tensa and the pars flaccida of the TM.
    - *The pars tensa*
      The fibrous layer of the pars tensa is attached to the malleus handle and to the tympanic bone and consists of two layers of densely packed collagenous fibers; one is oriented radially and another one oriented circularly [9, 10].
      - *Radial fibrous layers (stratum radiatum)* are attached to the manubrium and radiate outward to the annulus.
      - *Circular fibrous layer (stratum circulare)* is medial to the radial layer and has its fibers arranged concentrically and insert on the manubrium.
    - The pars flaccida
      The lamina propria of the pars flaccida is composed of small amount of elastic and collagenous fibers with no special arrangement and gradually passes into the dermis of the meatal skin [11].

Blood Supply of the Tympanic Membrane

- *Inner surface of the tympanic membrane*
  The TM is supplied by a vascular circle formed by the *anterior tympanic artery* branch from the internal maxillary artery and from the stylomastoid branch of the posterior auricular artery (Fig. 2.9).

- *Outer surface of the tympanic membrane*
  The tympanic membrane is supplied by the arteria manubrii having origin from the deep auricular branch of the internal maxillary artery.

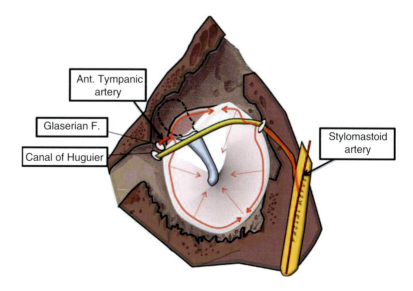

Fig. 2.9 Medial view of a left tympanic membrane showing tympanic membrane vascularization

Ant. Tympanic artery

Glaserian F.

Canal of Huguier

Stylomastoid artery

Nerves of the Tympanic Membrane

The membrane receives its innervations from the auriculotemporal branch of the mandibular nerve (CN V3), the tympanic branch of the glossopharyngeal nerve (CN IX), and the auricular branch of the vagus (CN X).

Clinical Application

Tympanic Membrane Retraction Pockets

- *Pars flaccida retraction pockets*
  The pars flaccida is the most common area of TM retraction pockets because it is the weakest part of the TM. Two reasons stand behind this weakness:
  1. Sparse amount of unorganized fibres in its lamina propria
  2. Direct insertion of the skin of the pars flaccida on the scutum in the absence of the combination annulus-sulcus, which acts like a ligament stabilizing the insertion of the TM to the surrounding bone [12]
- *Pars tensa retraction pockets*
  Pars tensa retraction pockets are more common in its posterosuperior part. Three reasons stand behind this fact:
  1. This part of the TM is more vascularized and thus more vulnerable to inflammation, which leads to secretion of collagenase and destruction of collagen fibers. This renders this part of the TM atrophic and prone to retraction in case of middle ear negative pressure.
  2. The middle fibrous layer of the posterosuperior part lacks a well-developed circular fibrous layer.
  3. The weak annulus insertion on the tympanic ring because of a shallow sulcus at this level [4].

  In contrary, the anterosuperior quadrant of the TM is less prone to retraction because of its strong insertion into the sulcus, the better arrangement of its circular fibers and the presence of the anterior malleal ligament acting as a support [4].

2.2 Inferior Wall (Jugular Wall)

2.2.1 Embryology of the Inferior Wall

The inferior wall of the middle ear develops between the 21st and the 31st gestational week, from the fusion of the tympanic bone and the petrosal bone. The fusion of these two bones, at 24th gestational week, closes the hypotympanum incompletely and leaves a persistent hypotympanic fissure, which houses the inferior tympanic canaliculus. The inferior tympanic canaliculus transmits the Jacobson's branch of the glossopharyngeal nerve and the inferior tympanic artery to the middle ear [13] (see Fig. 1.2) (see Sect. 1.1.1).

2.2.1.1 Development of the Jugular Bulb After Birth

The jugular bulb, absent at birth, is a dynamic structure which develops after the age of 2 years and reaches its definite size in adulthood. Children younger than 2 years old do not demonstrate the bulbous enlargement typical of the jugular bulb. The upward forces and the hemodynamic changes that accompany prone position lead to the bulbous enlargement typical of the adult jugular bulb. An erect posture, as opposed to the "fetal" or lying-down positions maintained in utero and in neonates, results in an ascending negative pulse wave originating from the heart and traversing upward to strike the jugular sinus at the jugular foramen. This phenomenon is responsible of the expansion of the jugular bulb [14].

Because the left brachiocephalic vein is relatively longer than the right one, it may dissipate the energy of the venous pulsation generated from the heart and consequently explain the development of a larger jugular bulb on the right side.

The absence of the jugular bulb at birth and its development in early infancy suggest that jugular bulb abnormalities are acquired rather than congenital and thus may progress with time to expand into the adjacent structures.

The venous blood flow dynamics may ultimately determine the variations in final size and position of the jugular bulb [14].

Fig. 2.10 Right ear after transcanal hypotympanotomy and dissection of the vertical portion of internal carotid artery (*VICA*) and the jugular bulb (*JB*), notice the emergence of the Jacobson's nerve (*J*) between the VICA and the JB and its relation to the round window (*RW*); also notice the relation of the horizontal portion of the internal carotid artery (*HICA*) and the Eustachian tube (*ET*); the HICA lies in the medial wall of the Eustachian tube

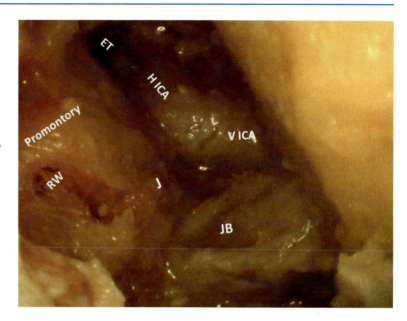

2.2.2   The Inferior Wall Anatomy

The floor of the middle ear cavity is narrow and consists of a thin plate of bone that separates the middle ear from the jugular bulb posteriorly and the internal carotid artery anteriorly. Between the carotid artery and the jugular bulb near the medial wall, there is a small canal, the inferior tympanic canaliculus, which transmits the Jacobson's nerve, branch of the glossopharyngeal nerve (CN IX), and the inferior tympanic artery (Fig. 2.10).

The surface of this wall may show irregularities due to the overlying pneumatized cells. In the posterior part of the floor is the root of the styloid process which gives rise to a bony eminence, the styloid eminence.

2.2.2.1   The Jugular Bulb

The jugular bulb connects the sigmoid sinus to the internal jugular vein.

It lies in the jugular fossa, an oval hollowed area at the internal and inferior surface of the petrous pyramid. The jugular bulb inhabits the posterior and largest compartment of the jugular foramen. The IX, X, and XI cranial nerves pass the skull base with this venous system.

The jugular bulb communicates with the cavernous sinus through the inferior petrosal sinus.

The jugular bulb dome lies at the floor of the middle ear cavity below the labyrinth and medial to the mastoid segment of the facial nerve.

It is variably positioned in relation to the hypotympanum, and its distance from the facial nerve laterally and the labyrinth superiorly is variable (Fig. 2.11). The distance from the jugular bulb to the posterior semicircular canal superiorly ranges from 0 to 10 mm (mean, 4 mm). The distance from the jugular bulb to the facial nerve laterally ranges from 0 to 12 mm (mean, 7 mm) [15].

Surgical Application
Retrofacial Approach to the Middle Ear
Retrofacial approach to the middle ear is done by drilling the area between the facial nerve laterally, the jugular bulb inferiorly and medially, and the ampulla of the posterior semicircular canal superiorly. This approach can provide a good access to the hypotympanum and the related structures without transposing the facial nerve or taking down the posterior external auditory canal wall. In cases with a high and lateral jugular bulb, this approach could not be done easily [15] (Fig. 2.12).

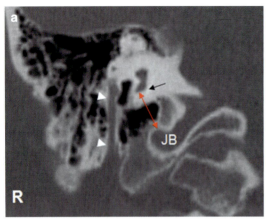
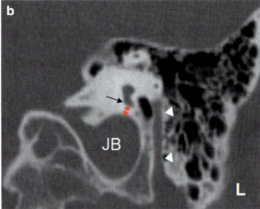

Fig. 2.11 Coronal computed tomographic reconstruction on the mastoid segment of the facial nerve (*arrowheads*) on both ears and the relation to the jugular bulb (*JB*) and the posterior semicircular canal (PSCC) (*black arrow*):

(**a**) On the right side (*R*), small jugular bulb (*JB*) with a large distance (*red arrow*) to the PSCC. (**b**) On the left side (*L*), huge JB with a short distance (*red arrow*) to the PSCC

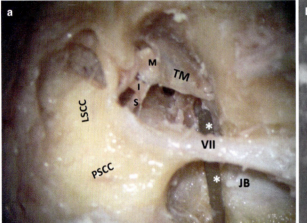
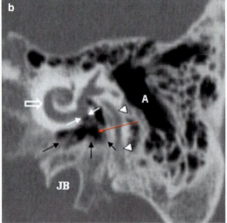

Fig. 2.12 (**a**) Retrofacial approach in a left ear hypotympanum. (*) surgical instrument; *VII* mastoid segment of the facial nerve, *JB* jugular bulb, *TM* tympanic membrane, *M* malleus, *I* incus, *S* stapes, *LSCC* lateral semicircular canal, *PSCC* posterior semicircular canal. (**b**) Sagittal oblique reconstruction of a computed tomography show-

ing the retrofacial hypotympanotomy approach (*red arrow*). Mastoid segment of the VII nerve (*arrowheads*), hypotympanic air cells (*black arrows*), round window membrane (between the *white arrows*), basal turn of the cochlea (*empty arrow*). *A* antrum, *JB* jugular bulb

Clinical Application

Jugular Bulb Anomalies

A high jugular bulb (HJB) is a condition in which the jugular bulb dome rides above the tympanic annulus. A HJB has an intact sigmoid plate which separates it from the middle ear cavity. If the sigmoid plate is deficient, the bulb protrudes into the middle ear cavity; this situation is called a dehiscent jugular bulb (JBD) (Fig. 2.13).

A HJB or JBD manifests as a pulsatile tinnitus and appears like a posteroinferior retrotympanic blue mass on otoscopic examination. Injury of a JBD during tympanomeatal flap elevation results in profuse bleeding [16, 17].

The incidence of high JB ranges from 5 to 20 % and that of JBD ranges from 1 to 10 % [17].

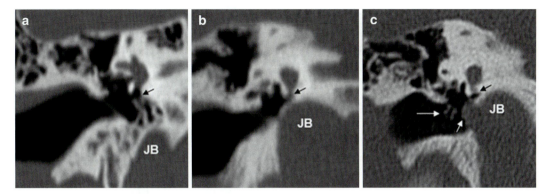

Fig. 2.13 (**a**) Coronal computed tomographic view on a right ear with a normal jugular bulb (*JB*), round window recess (*black arrow*). (**b**) High riding JB obliterating the round window recess (*black arrow*). (**c**) JB diverticula (*small white arrow*), reaching the round window recess (*black arrow*). Notice the transtympanic tube in place (*long white arrow*)

Fig. 2.14 15.5-mm human embryo coronal section showing the laterohyale (*arrow*) covering facial nerve rudiment (*), in connection with the Reichert's cartilage (*R*). Hematoxylin-eosin staining

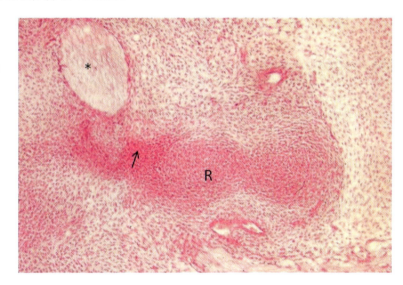

2.3 Posterior Wall

2.3.1 Embryology of the Posterior Wall

The posterior wall develops from the Reichert's cartilage. The facial nerve develops in a groove on the otic capsule. By the 20th week, the facial canal is better defined by fibrous tissue laterally as the otic capsule ossifies medially. Reichert's cartilage persists as a cartilage bar interposed between the otic capsule and the facial nerve medially and the tympanic annulus laterally [18]. Ossification starts in this cartilage bar and continues in the mesenchyme both medial and lateral to this cartilage bar, forming the facial canal and the posterior wall of the middle ear cavity. The cartilage remnant of Reichert's bar frequently persists to the time of birth, ossifying separately from the surrounding mesenchyme. The first cartilaginous wall of the facial canal is the laterohyale connected primitively with the interhyale, rudiment of the stapedial tendon (Fig. 2.14).

2.3.2 Posterior Wall Anatomy

The posterior wall is the highest wall of the middle ear and measures about 14 mm. It is formed essentially by the petrous bone. The posterior

Fig. 2.15 A medial view of a left middle ear showing the posterior wall composed of an inferior closed part separating the middle ear from the mastoid and a superior open part, the aditus ad antrum, which connects the middle ear to the mastoid. Notice that the floor of the aditus houses the fossa incudis (*FI*), which lodges the short process of the incus (*SPI*)

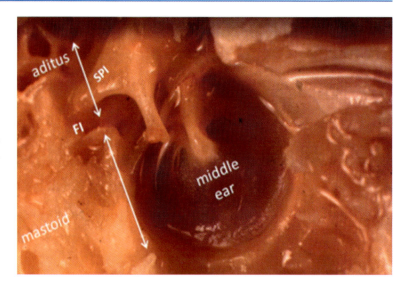

wall separates the middle ear from the mastoid air cells, except at the area of the aditus ad antrum, where it is deficient and permits communication between the attic and the mastoid antrum.

The posterior wall can be divided into two distinct parts: the upper third which corresponds to the *aditus ad antrum* and represents the posterior limit of the epitympanum and the lower two thirds which correspond to the posterior wall of the retrotympanum.

The two parts are separated by the incudal buttress which is a compact bone that runs from the tympanic ring laterally to the lateral semicircular canal medially. It houses the *incudal fossa* in its superior surface which lodges the short process of the incus (Fig. 2.15).

2.3.2.1 The Upper Part: The Aditus Ad Antrum

The aditus ad antrum connects the epitympanum of the middle ear to the mastoid antrum posteriorly. The aditus is of a triangular shape with dimensions of 4×4×4 mm height, length, and width (see Sect. 5.2.3 and Fig. 5.17).

2.3.2.2 The Lower Part: The Posterior Wall of the Tympanum

The posterior wall of the tympanum is a complete bony wall and bridges the bony annulus tympanicus to the bony labyrinth. It is the extension of the styloid eminence upward to the pyramidal eminence and to the level of the fossa

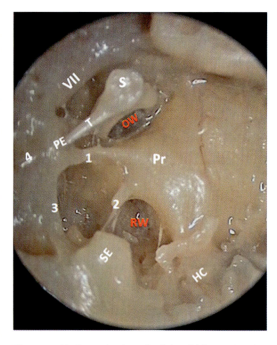

Fig. 2.16 Endoscopic view of a right middle ear showing the different ridges of the posterior wall. *1* ponticulus, *2* subiculum, *3* pyramidal ridge, *4* chordal ridge, *PE* pyramidal eminence, *SE* styloid eminence, *OW* oval window, *RW* round window, *S* stapes, *T* stapedial tendon, *Pr* promontory, *HC* hypotympanic cells, *VII* facial nerve

incudis. It houses the vertical segment of the facial nerve.

This wall is wider above than below and presents three eminences directed anteriorly, five bony ridges, and four sinuses delimiting the retrotympanum spaces (Fig. 2.16).

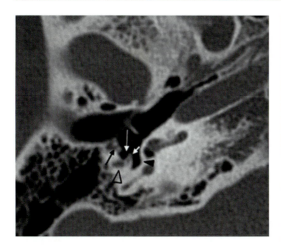

Fig. 2.17 Transversal computed tomography of the posterior wall of the cavity. From lateral to medial: chordal eminence (*black arrow*), facial recess (*long white arrow*), facial nerve (*empty arrowhead*), pyramidal eminence (*short white arrow*), sinus tympani (*black arrowhead*)

Posterior Wall Eminences

The posterior wall presents three bony eminences: the pyramidal, chordal, and styloid eminences. These three eminences altogether form what is called the *styloid complex,* which is a derivative of the superior portion of the second branchial arch.

- *The pyramidal eminence*
  The pyramidal eminence is situated at the center of the posterior wall immediately behind the oval window; it is about 2 mm height. Its base is fused with the canal of the facial nerve. It lodges the body of the stapedial muscle and its apex gives passage to the stapedial tendon. The pyramidal eminence communicates with the facial bony canal by a minute aperture which transmits the stapedial branch of the facial nerve (Fig. 2.17).
- *The chordal eminence*
  The chordal eminence is situated lateral to the pyramidal eminence and 1 mm medial to the tympanic membrane. The chordal eminence shows a foramen: the *iter chordæ posterius* through which the chorda tympani nerve gains access to the middle ear cavity (Fig. 2.17).
- *The styloid eminence*
  The styloid eminence or Politzer eminence is a recognized smoothed elevation at the inferior part of the posterior wall; it represents the base of the styloid process.

During transcanal hypotympanotomy, the styloid eminence represents a very important landmark for the facial nerve; the styloid eminence is always anterior to the facial nerve and represents the posterior limit of safe drilling in the posterior part of the hypotympanum.

Posterior Wall Ridges

We can identify in the posterior wall five bony ridges which connect the eminences with each other and with the promontory.

- *The chordal ridge of Proctor*
  The chordal ridge runs laterally and transversally from the pyramidal eminence to fuse with the chordal eminence.
- *The pyramidal ridge*
  The pyramidal ridge is very prominent. It runs inferiorly from the base of the pyramidal eminence to the styloid eminence. It could be absent.
- *The styloid ridge*
  The styloid ridge connects the styloid prominence to the chordal eminence.
- *The ponticulus*
  The ponticulus is a central structure in the retrotympanum. It is a bony ridge extending from the pyramidal process to the promontory. There are two different variants of the ponticulus:
  - Complete ponticulus: when the ponticulus is completely formed and extends from the pyramidal process to the promontory area. In this case the ponticulus represents the superior frontier of the sinus tympani and separates it from the posterior sinus.
  - Incomplete ponticulus: in this case the ponticulus does not connect with the pyramidal process making the sinus tympani and the posterior sinus one confluent sinus.
- *The subiculum*
  The subiculum is a smooth bony projection that is situated posterior to the promontory and extends inferiorly from the posterior lip of the round window niche towards the styloid eminence. Therefore, it intervenes between the sinus tympani superiorly and the round window inferiorly.

Posterior Wall Spaces

The posterior wall bony eminences and ridges divide the posterior wall into four different spaces that are completely separated from the mastoid cavity (see Sect. 4.4).

2.4   Superior Wall (The Tegmen)

The superior wall of the middle ear cavity is a plate of bone that separates the middle ear cavity from the overlying middle cranial fossa dura and temporal lobe of cerebrum. The integrity of the tegmen is essential to avoid spread of infection from the middle ear to the intracranial cavity, as well as to prevent herniation of the brain into the middle ear.

2.4.1   Superior Wall Development

The superior wall forms from the fusion of two horizontal plates, a small lateral plate (*horizontal process*) derived from the squamous bone and a large medial plate (*tegmental process*) derived from the otic capsule of the petrous bone. The lateral plate shows membranous ossification, whereas the medial one shows endochondral ossification (see Fig. 1.2) (see Sect. 1.1.1).

At the line of fusion of both plates, a bony log is formed and is called the tignum transversum that is the major supporting element of the tegmen. The tignum transversum extends anteriorly to the Glaserian fissure and then beaks medially to form the so-called cog [19].

Delayed or incomplete ossification of the tegmen may lead to tegmen defects observed in childhood or early, with possible meningocele or spontaneous CSF fistula (Fig. 2.18).

> **Clinical Implications**
> **Middle Ear Meningoencephalocele**
> Middle ear meningoencephalocele is a herniation of brain tissue through a bony defect into the middle ear. Middle cranial fossa meningoencephaloceles are the most common, and this is related to tegmen tympani dehiscence under the weight of the temporal brain lobe and CSF pulsations effect [20, 21]. The most frequent bony defect in the tegmen tympani is in the region next to the geniculate ganglion [22] (see Fig. 2.18).
> Posterior cranial fossa meningoencephalocele into the middle ear is rare.

2.4.2   Superior Wall Anatomy

The tegmen is a thin bony plate that forms the roof of the middle ear cavity and separates it from the overlying temporal lobe. The part of the tegmen overlying the Eustachian tube is called *tegmen tubari*, the part overlying the tympanic cavity is called the *tegmen tympani,* and that overlying the mastoid antrum is called the *tegmen antri*.

The superior surface of the tegmen forms part of middle cranial fossa floor and is covered by the dura; the inferior surface of the tegmen is lined

Fig. 2.18 Coronal computed tomography of the right ear showing in (**a**) congenital dehiscence of the tegmen (*arrowhead*); (**b**) herniation of endocranial tissue of the middle fossa through a congenital dehiscence of the tegmen (*between the long arrows*), laterally to the geniculate ganglion (*), reaching the ossicles (*short arrow*)

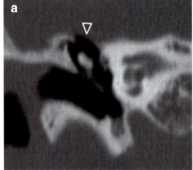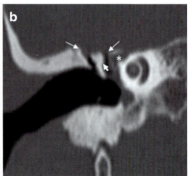

Fig. 2.19 A sagittal cut of the temporal bone, showing the superior wall of a left middle ear (*ME*). *MCF* middle cranial fossa, *ET* Eustachian tube

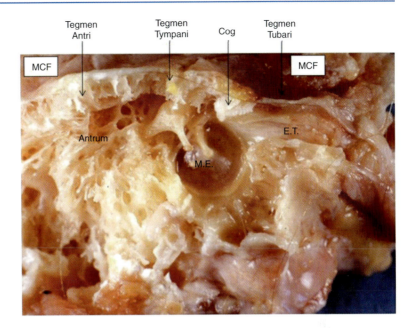

by middle ear mucosa. The tegmen separates the cerebrospinal fluid superiorly from the air of the middle ear inferiorly [23] (Fig. 2.19).

The tegmen tympani is formed from two unequal bony plates. The largest medial portion develops from the tegmental plate of the petrous bone, and the smaller lateral portion develops from the horizontal plate of the squamous bone (Fig. 2.20).

The suture line between these two plates is known as the internal petrosquamous suture.

In newborns, this suture is not ossified and is filled with connective tissue; it does not close until adulthood [24]. In adults, the dura of the middle cranial fossa is tightly adherent to this suture; sharp dissection may be required for elevation of the dura at this level during middle cranial fossa approach.

In the middle ear surface of the petrosquamous fissure serves as a point of attachment to the superior malleal and superior incudal ligaments.

In the anterior attic, the tegmen is formed completely by the tegmental plate of the petrous bone. In the posterior attic and in the antrum, the horizontal plate of the squamous bone contributes to the formation of the tegmen tympani [22] (Fig. 2.20).

At the level of fusion between the tegmental plate and anterior limit of the horizontal plate, the cog appears (Fig. 2.20). The cog is a 0.5-mm long transversal hard and dense bony crest situated 1–2 mm anterior to the malleus head and heading vertically towards the cochleariform process. Its medial part may eventually prolong to reach the cochleariform process [25, 26].

2.4.2.1 Supportive Mechanisms of the Tegmen

As described above, the tignum transversum is the major supporting element of the tegmen. In addition to the tignum transversum, the carrying capacity of the tegmen depends on the lateral and medial processes of the tignum as well. The tignum transversum and the medial and lateral processes establish a structure similar to the nervation of a leaf. This aspect of a nervation assures an evenly distributed mechanical support for the thin and eventually perforated plate of the tegmen. Thus, the resistivity of a thin tegmen against the weight of the temporal lobe and cerebrospinal pulsations is determined more by the complete structure of the described network of the bone rather than by the thickness of the plate [19] (Fig. 2.21).

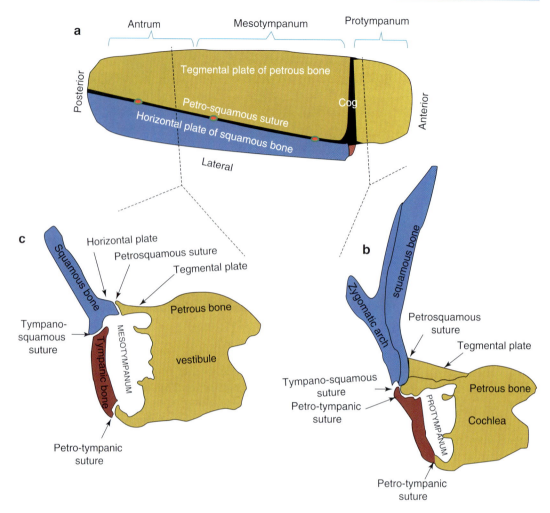

Fig. 2.20 (**a**) Superior view of the tegmen from the middle cranial fossa demonstrates the setup of the tegmen tympani formed by two distinct bony plates of the temporal bone, with the horizontal process of the squamous part laterally and the tegmental process of the petrous part medially. Both plates meet at the petrosquamous fissure. (**b**) Section made through the protympanum shows that the roof of the protympanum is built up only by the tegmental process. (**c**) Section made through the mesotympanum showing that the squamous part contributes to the formation of the tegmen tympani in this area

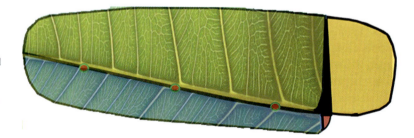

Fig. 2.21 The carrying capacity of the tegmen depends on the tignum transversum (*black line*) and its associated lateral and medial processes; these together establish structures similar to the nervation of a leaf

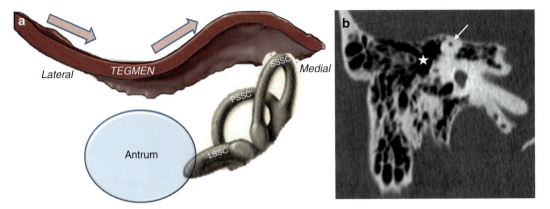

Fig. 2.22 (**a**) 3D image of the tegmen in the coronal plane. The tegmen slopes down above the antrum and then goes up to cover the superior semicircular canal. *SSSC* superior semicircular canal, *PSSC* posterior semicircular canal, *LSCC* lateral semicircular canal. (**b**) Computed tomography of a right ear showing the shape variation of the tegmen relatively to the antrum (*) and the superior arch of the SCCC (*white arrow*)

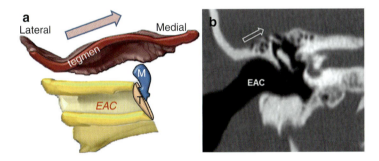

Fig. 2.23 (**a**) 3D Image in the coronal plane showing the relationship between the tegmen and the bony external ear canal. Notice that the tegmen rises up as we move medially (*arrow*). *EAC* external auditory canal, *T* tympanic membrane, *M* malleus. (**b**) Coronal computed tomography of a right ear showing the slope of the tegmen (*arrow*) upwards in relation to the superior wall of the external auditory canal (*EAC*) in lateral-to-medial direction

2.4.2.2 Surgical Anatomy of the Tegmen

Mastoid surgery and atticotomy require complete conservation of the tegmental plate.

Since the tegmen shows a variable shape and inclination and because the dura and the arachnoid are closely adherent to the bone in the middle fossa region, iatrogenic injuries by drilling could lead to cerebrospinal fluid leak, pneumocephalus, brain herniation, or cerebral abscess. Thus, a thorough knowledge of the tegmen slopes as well as its relationship with the external auditory canal is essential for a safe and successful attico-mastoid surgery. The tegmen is not a simple horizontal plane, but it is an irregular plate of bone with ondulating slopes.

There are two distinct slopes in the configuration of the tegmen: one is from lateral to medial and a second one is from posterior to anterior direction.

Lateral-to-Medial Slope

In the lateral-to-medial direction, the tegmen presents an inferiorly directed hang before heading up to its highest point above the superior semicircular canal (Fig. 2.22). This shape of hanging down laterally and rising up medially exists throughout the whole course of the tegmen as in its posterior or in its anterior part [27].

Over the external auditory canal (Fig. 2.23), the majority of the population has a narrower distance laterally than medially [27].

Posterior-to-Anterior Slope

In the sagittal plane the tegmen makes also a slope in a posterior to anterior direction and becomes close to the superior part of the external auditory canal [27]. The tegmen is higher posteriorly by about 1–10 mm than anteriorly (Fig. 2.24).

Surgical Application

During mastoid dissection anteriorly it is recommended to start first inferiorly, then progress back around superiorly. Therefore, while approaching the superior wall of the external auditory canal and knowing that the dura hangs down laterally, the surgeons' drill must work from medial to lateral to avoid lowering or injuring the canal wall or hitting the dura. The tegmen can be easily damaged laterally where the dura is low lying. Also this lateral overhang can obscure the disease tissues hidden medially.

In addition, if the medial level of the dura is wrongly expected to be at the same lower lateral level, the drilling may wrongly progress much lower medially and could traumatize the lateral semicircular canal or facial canal [27].

The sagittal plane is especially relevant when extending the drilling from the antrum to the attic region anteriorly: the tegmen slopes inferiorly as the drilling progresses anteriorly. One should expect a much lower dura anteriorly at the level of root of the zygoma; this is of most concern during anterior epitympanic recess approach (Fig. 2.23).

The space available to work between the EAC wall and the dural plate in canal wall-up attico-mastoidectomy is smaller than posteriorly. Basically this finding confirms that the root of zygoma is a surgically challenging area, especially when approaching the anterior attic with conservation of the ossicular chain in place. In this procedure care must be taken not to penetrate the external canal wall nor to injure the dura in a canal wall-up technique.

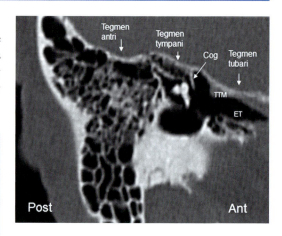

Fig. 2.24 Sagittal reconstruction of a computed tomography of a temporal bone showing the different parts of the tegmen and the cog. Note that the tegmen slopes downwards from posterior to anterior. *TTM* tensor tympani muscle, *ET* Eustachian tube

---

2.5 Anterior Wall (Carotid Wall)

The anterior wall separates the middle ear cavity from the petrous carotid artery canal. It houses the tympanic orifice of the Eustachian tube.

2.5.1 Anterior Wall Development

The development of the anterior wall and the protympanum is in close relationship to that of the carotid canal and the auditory tube. The anterior wall arises completely from the petrous bone.

After the development of the otic capsule at the 16th week of gestation, multiple plates extend laterally from the otic capsule around the developing tubotympanic recess and ICA to build up almost the entire protympanum (Fig. 2.25). The tympanic bone forms the posterior border of the lateral wall of the protympanum [28]. In the protympanum, the bone appears in the 18th week.

The developmental junction between petrous and tympanic bones is marked by the petrotympanic fissure, or Glaserian fissure, which continues laterally into the tympanosquamous fissure.

2.5.1.1 Development of the Carotid Canal

The development of the carotid canal has a close relationship with the internal carotid artery (ICA)

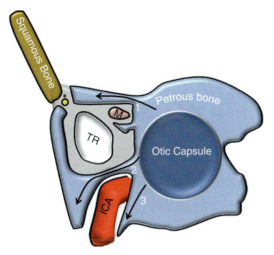

Fig. 2.25 Schematic drawing of the developing protympanum and its surroundings in the frontal plane (34-week-old fetus). The walls of the protympanum are built up by several processes of the petrous bone: the tegmental plate (*1*) forming the roof, the superior lamina of the carotid canal (*2*) and the inferior lamina of carotid canal (*3*) forming the inferomedial wall. The medial wall of the protympanum is created by the promontory itself. *M* tensor tympani muscle, *TR* tubotympanic recess, *ICA* internal carotid artery, * chorda tympani

development. In the early embryonic period, the ICA lies on the anterior part of the cartilaginous otic capsule; ossification of the otic capsule that starts in the 18th week produces two plates around the ICA, the superior and the inferior plate. At birth, the plates of the carotid canal have enclosed the ICA in a bony channel in the medial wall of the protympanum [28] (Fig. 2.25).

If the ICA is not directly beside the otic capsule, the bony canal of the ICA will be absent [29].

Consequently ICA dehiscence encountered in children is the result of incomplete fusion of the superior and inferior bony plates of the carotid canal. Furthermore, agenesis of the internal carotid artery is associated to an absence of the carotid canal [30] (see Sect. 3.5.1.2).

2.5.2   Anterior Wall Anatomy

The anterior wall of the tympanic cavity is very narrow because the medial and lateral walls of the middle ear cavity converge anteriorly in an acute angle. The anterior wall is formed entirely from the petrous bone and can be divided into three portions: the lower, the middle, and the upper portion (Fig. 2.26).

2.5.2.1   The Lower Portion

The lower portion of the anterior wall is the largest portion and represents the anterior wall of the hypotympanum. It is a thin plate of bone that separates the middle ear cavity from the vertical segment of the petrous carotid artery. This bony plate has two tiny openings for the

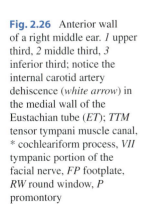

Fig. 2.26 Anterior wall of a right middle ear. *1* upper third, *2* middle third, *3* inferior third; notice the internal carotid artery dehiscence (*white arrow*) in the medial wall of the Eustachian tube (*ET*); *TTM* tensor tympani muscle canal, * cochleariform process, *VII* tympanic portion of the facial nerve, *FP* footplate, *RW* round window, *P* promontory

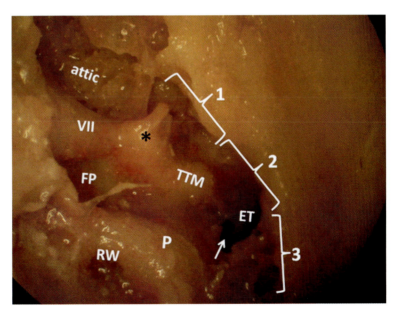

caroticotympanic nerves: the upper opening transmits the superior caroticotympanic nerve and the inferior opening transmits the inferior caroticotympanic nerve. These nerves have origin from the pericarotid sympathetic chain; they transmit sympathetic fibers coming from the superior cervical ganglia to the tympanic plexus of the middle ear.

2.5.2.2 The Middle Portion

The middle portion of the anterior wall corresponds to the protympanum. The middle portion has two tunnels placed one below the other: the upper tunnel transmits the tensor tympani muscle, and the lower tunnel corresponds to the bony portion of the Eustachian tube. A thin horizontal plate of bone, the septum canalis musculotubari, separates these two tunnels from each other.

- The semicanal for the tensor tympani (semicanalis m. tensoris tympani) is cylindrical and lies beneath the tegmen tympani. It extends to join the cochleariform process.
- The septum canalis musculotubarii passes posteriorly below the tensor tympani semicanal; it expands above the anterior end of the oval window and terminates by curving laterally forming a pulley, the cochleariform process, over which the tendon of the tensor tympani muscle passes [31].
- The bony portion of the Eustachian tube: is situated below the septum canalis (see Sect. 7.2.1).

2.5.2.3 The Upper Portion

The upper portion of the anterior wall corresponds to the root of the zygoma which represents the anterior wall of the epitympanum.

2.5.2.4 The Carotid Artery and the Anterior Wall

The carotid artery enters the temporal bone through the carotid foramen. It ascends vertically in the anterior wall of the hypotympanum and in the medial wall of the bony Eustachian tube at the area just beneath the cochlea (the vertical segment); then it turns anteromedially at almost a right angle towards the petrous apex, forming the horizontal segment anteroinferiorly to the cochlea (Figs. 2.10 and 2.27).

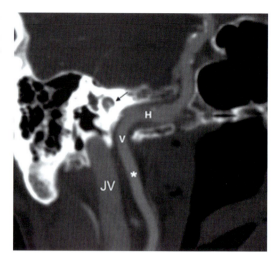

Fig. 2.27 CT Angio-scan of the supra-aortic right vessels, with a sagittal oblique reconstruction, showing the trajectory of the internal carotid artery (*) with its vertical (*V*) and horizontal (*H*) segment. Note the relationship to the basal turn of the cochlea (*black arrow*). *JV* jugular vein

The Vertical Segment of the Petrous Carotid Canal

The vertical segment of the petrous carotid canal is 5.0–12.5 mm in height and 4.0–7.5 mm in diameter.

The vertical segment is separated from the middle ear cavity by a thin plate of bone of about 0.25 mm. There is no difference in thickness between pediatric and adult subjects. A dehiscence of carotid canal is observed in about 5 % of temporal bones, usually located at the medial wall of the bony portion of Eustachian tube (Fig. 2.26).

The tympanic bone is anterolateral to the vertical segment [32]. The distance from the anterior margin of the tympanic annulus to the nearest point of carotid canal is about 5 mm [33].

The Horizontal Segment of the Petrous Carotid Canal

The horizontal segment of the petrous carotid canal is directed anteromedially by a path of 14.5–24 mm long and 4.5–7.0 mm in diameter [32]. The average distance between the carotid canal and the cochlea is about 1 mm near the basal turn, 2 mm near the middle turn, and 6 mm near the apical turn [34].

Fig. 2.28 Coronal reconstruction of a computed tomography of a left ear with (**a**) normal bony separation (*) between the cochlea and the internal carotid artery (*ICA*); (**b**) a dehiscent internal carotid artery (*white arrow*) into the basal turn of the cochlea

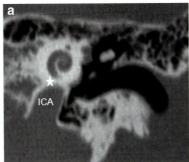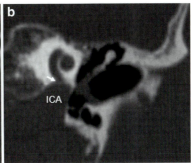

Surgical Implication

Rarely, there is partial absence of septation between the cochlea and the carotid canal. In these cases, preoperative imaging of the temporal bone shows the anatomical relationship between the cochlea and petrous carotid canal and may help prevent inadvertent penetration of the carotid canal during cochlear implant surgery (Fig. 2.28).

2.6 Medial Wall (Cochlear Wall)

The medial wall is formed mainly by the cochlear promontory in addition to several important structures: the tympanic segment of the facial nerve, the oval and the round windows, the tensor tympani canal, the cochleariform process, and the lateral semicircular canal.

2.6.1 Embryology of the Medial Wall Structures

2.6.1.1 Facial Nerve VII, Tympanic Segment (See Chap. 6)

The horizontal segment of the facial nerve is recognized by the sixth week when it passes between the developing membranous labyrinth and the primitive stapes [35]. By the eighth week, soon after the stapes blastema reaches the otic capsule, a sulcus forms within the lateral margin of the cartilaginous otic capsule, initiating the formation of the horizontal facial nerve canal; this groove forms by the tenth week. If this canal is deep and well formed, the facial nerve will be

"locked in" to its normal anatomic position against the otic capsule [35]. The facial nerve groove will begin to enclose the facial nerve in the 4th gestational month. Ossification of the canal is completed during or shortly after the first year of life [36].

2.6.1.2 Oval Window

The oval window is derived from the lateral surface of the otic capsule. Its development is related directly to the development of second branchial arch structures and most importantly the stapes and the facial nerve. As early as the fifth week, the blastemal mass of the stapes becomes recognizable as a ring-shaped structure around the stapedial artery. This rudimentary stapes grows medially, then contacts and indents the developing otic capsule at the future oval window during the seventh week. The mesenchyme in this depression fuses with the stapedial ring to form the stapes footplate [37, 38]. Once the base of the stapes has fully developed, dedifferentiation of the oval window cartilage occurs, and a rim of fibrous tissue forms to produce the annular ligament [36].

Clinical Implications

Oval Window Atresia

When the primitive stapes fails to fuse with the primitive vestibule, the oval window cannot develop, resulting in its congenital absence. One widely accepted explanation for the congenital absence of the oval window proposes that during the fifth and sixth weeks of gestation, the developing facial nerve becomes anteriorly displaced and interposed between the otic capsule and the stapes blastema. As a result, the contact between the stapes and the otic capsule is prevented; thus, the development of the oval window is not initiated [35, 39, 40]. An abnormal appearance of the stapes is often associated with congenital absence of the oval window.

In addition, a congenital absence of the oval window could be associated with different anomalies of the tympanic segment of the facial nerve canal such as a low-lying facial nerve relative to the oval window or a canal situated within or below the expected location of the oval window or a dehiscent large facial nerve [41].

Failure of development of the annular ligament results in congenital fixation of the stapes footplate.

2.6.1.3   Fissula Ante Fenestram

The fissula ante fenestram is part of the perilymphatic labyrinth and it is unique to humans. The fissula is first apparent in the ninth week (embryo of 34 mm) [42], as a strip of precartilage in the lateral wall of the cartilaginous otic capsule immediately anterior to the oval window. During the next 3 weeks, this extension of periotic tissue stretches as a connective tissue ribbon from the vestibule to the middle ear. The fissula continues to grow until mid-fetal life about 21st week, at which time the ossification of the otic capsule is almost completed (Fig. 2.29). The cartilage border that separates the connective tissue of the fissula from the bone of the otic capsule is gradually replaced by intrachondral bone.

Because of the metamorphosis of the lining cartilage rests, the fissula is thought to be the area of histological instability. Later in life the new bone-forming process may be enhanced and expand to become an active focus of otosclerosis [43].

2.6.1.4   Round Window

The round window area appears during the 11th week. By this time ossification has started in the otic capsule. During the ossification of the otic capsule, the round window niche is surrounded by a thickened ring of cartilage which isolates the round window mesenchyme from the ossifying otic capsule and prevents the ossification of the round window opening. Further differentiation of the cartilage ring forms the round window niche, and the round window membrane appears inside the niche with an epithelial layer of mucous membrane. Mesenchymal tissue left unabsorbed in the round window niche may form a separate outer membrane, closing off the actual niche.

When the cartilage ring does not develop, osseous obliteration will occur and lead to congenital round window atresia [44].

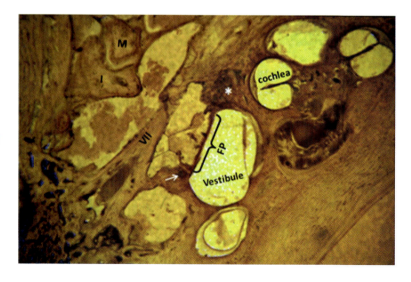

Fig. 2.29 Transverse cut of a left temporal bone of a 28-week-old embryo showing the fissula ante fenestram (*) in front of the footplate (*FP*) and the fissula post fenestram posterior to the footplate (*white arrow*). *VII* facial nerve, *I* incus, *M* malleus

Fig. 2.30 Endoscopic view of a left middle ear. *VII* tympanic facial nerve, * cochleariform process, *TTM* tensor tympani muscle, *RW* round window, *ET* Eustachian tube, *FP* footplate, *P* promontory, *HC* hypotympanic cells, *ST* sinus tympani, *Pon* ponticulus, *Sub* subiculum

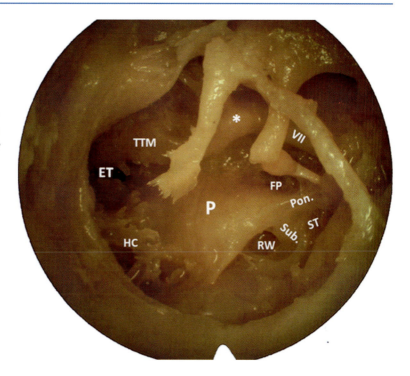

The ossification of the walls of the round window niche starts at the 16th week and is established by both membranous and endochondral ossification. However, related to the different degrees of this double ossification types, there will be a great variability in the phenotypes of the round window niche. Depending on the state of development of the upper and anterior walls of the niche, the plane of the opening of the round window niche can be horizontal, dorsal, or lateral.

2.6.2   Medial Wall Anatomy

The medial wall of the tympanic cavity separates the middle ear cleft from the adjacent inner ear. The canal of the tensor tympani muscle anteriorly and the tympanic Fallopian canal posteriorly are two landmarks that divide the medial wall into upper third part and lower two third part. The upper third forms the medial wall of the epitympanum and is demarcated posteriorly by the lateral semicircular canal (LSCC). The lower two-thirds form the medial wall of the

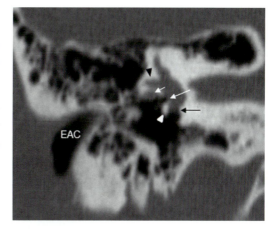

Fig. 2.31 Coronal computed tomographic reconstruction of a right ear. The medial wall of the middle ear cavity from upward to downwards: the lateral semicircular canal (*black arrowhead*), the tympanic facial nerve (*short white arrow*), the oval window (*long white arrow*), the round window (*black arrow*), promontory (*white arrowhead*), *EAC* external auditory canal

mesotympanum and include the cochlear promontory on the center, the oval window posterosuperiorly, and the round window posteroinferiorly (Figs. 2.30 and 2.31).

2.6.2.1 Tensor Tympanic Muscle Bony Canal and the Cochleariform Process

The semicanal of the tensor tympani muscle (semicanalis m. tensoris tympani) is cylindrical and extends from the protympanum on to the labyrinthine wall of the tympanic cavity and ends immediately in front of the oval window niche.

The medial wall of the tympanic cavity is marked by a slightly curved bone protruding laterally called the cochleariform process which is situated anterosuperior to the oval window and just inferior to the tympanic segment of the facial nerve. It represents the posterior end of the bony canal of the TTM. This curved projection of bone is concave anteriorly, and it houses the tendon of the tensor tympani muscle. The tendon turns laterally and attaches at the medial aspect of the handle of the malleus.

> **Surgical Pearl**
> The cochleariform process is a highly important anatomical and surgical landmark to identify the facial nerve and the oval window in invasive pathologies (Fig. 2.32).

2.6.2.2 Facial Nerve Canal

The prominence of facial nerve canal is an important anatomical structure present in the upper part of the medial wall of the mesotympanum. This nerve canal runs obliquely above the promontory and above the oval window in an anteroposterior direction from above the cochleariform process anteriorly down below and medial to the dome of the lateral semicircular canal. It presents its second genu at the turning point between the horizontal tympanic portion and the vertically descending mastoid portion in the posterior wall of the tympanic cavity.

In the medial wall the bony canal of VII could be dehiscent to leave the VII only covered with a submucosa or even prolapsing lying over the oval window (see Chap. 6). This situation is highly at risk during middle ear surgery. Even infections of the middle ear mucosa can cause facial nerve palsy in patients with an exposed facial nerve (Figs. 2.31 and 2.32).

2.6.2.3 Lateral Semicircular Canal

The region above the level of the facial nerve canal forms the medial wall of the attic. The dome of the lateral semicircular canal extends a little lateral to the facial canal and is the most

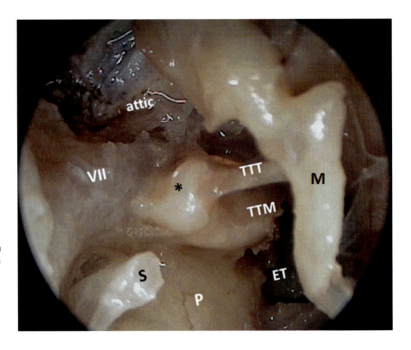

Fig. 2.32 Endoscopic view of a right middle ear through a posterior tympanotomy showing the tympanic segment of the facial nerve (*VII*) and its relationship with the cochleariform process (*) and stapes (*S*). *TTM* tensor tympani muscle, *TTT* tensor tympani tendon, *P* promontory, *ET* Eustachian tube, *M* malleus

Fig. 2.33 Medial wall of the attic. *LSCC* lateral semicircular canal, *VII* facial nerve, *M* malleus, *PIL* posterior incudal ligament, *SIL* superior incudal ligament, *SML* superior malleal ligament, * incudal fossa

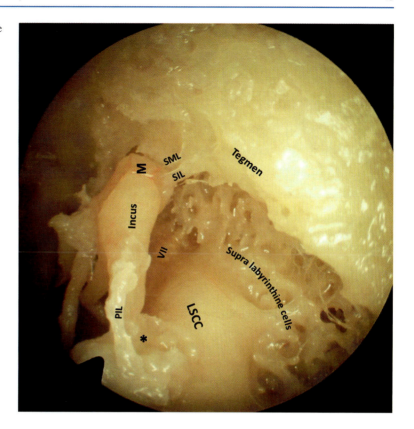

prominent structure of the posterior portion of the epitympanum (Figs. 2.31 and 2.33).

2.6.2.4   The Cochlear Promontory

The promontory is a prominent eminence occupying most of the central portion of the medial wall of the middle ear and lodges between the oval and round windows. This projection represents the underlying basal turn of the cochlea (Fig. 2.34a).

The promontory surface is grooved to accommodate the branches of the tympanic plexus (Jacobson's nerve), which enters the temporal bone through the tympanic canaliculus, just anterior to the jugular foramen.

Surgical Pearl

The basal turn of the human cochlea is a bony canal. The least covered portion is located behind the apex of the promontory. The lower half of the basal turn of the cochlea can be approached from the facial recess or external auditory canal during cochlear implantation. The second and third turn of the cochlea are also approachable from the tympanic cavity; nevertheless, to be able to reveal the second and third turns fully, the tensor tympani muscle and the semicanal must be completely removed (Fig. 2.34).

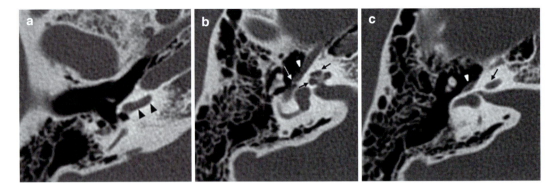

Fig. 2.34 Transversal computed tomography of a right ear. The medial wall of the middle ear in relation to (**a**) the basal turn of the cochlea (*arrowheads*). (**b**) The second turn of the cochlea (*black arrows*), the tensor tympani muscle (*white arrowhead*), the cochleariform process (*white arrow*). (**c**) The highest level of the cochlea (*arrow*), facial nerve (*arrowhead*)

2.6.2.5 The Oval Window Niche

The oval window niche (fenestra vestibuli) is located in the medial wall of the posterior part of the mesotympanum behind and above the promontory inferior to the facial nerve canal.

The oval window niche is limited anteriorly and superiorly by the cochleariform process and posteriorly by the ponticulus, sinus tympani, and pyramidal eminence. It is situated in a depression called the fossula vestibuli where its depth depends on the facial nerve position and the variable prominence of the promontory (Fig. 2.30).

It is a kidney-shaped opening leading to the vestibule of the inner ear. The long diameter of the oval window is horizontal and its convex border is directed upward. It is closed by the footplate of the stapes which is rounded by the annular ligament. The dimensions of the oval window average 3.25 mm long and 1.75 mm wide.

Fissula Ante Fenestram

The fissula ante fenestram is considered as an appendage of the perilymphatic labyrinth; it is a strip of periotic connective tissue extending from the vestibule just anterior to the oval window through an irregular still-like space in the bony otic capsule to join the mucoperiosteum of the tympanic cavity below the pulley of the tensor tympani muscle. Usually it is obliterated by fibrous tissue and immature cartilage (Fig. 2.35).

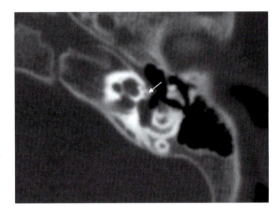

Fig. 2.35 Transversal computed tomography showing the normal appearance of the fissula ante fenestram (*white arrow*) in a child

Fissula Post Fenestram

This is an evagination of the periotic tissue into the otic capsule just posterior to the oval window at a point about one third of the way between the window and the non-ampullated end of the lateral semicircular canal.

> **Clinical Application**
>
> In cases of otosclerosis, the oval window can be the site of different degrees of invasion, ranging from a typical focal anteroinferior thickening to a complete obliteration (Fig. 2.36).

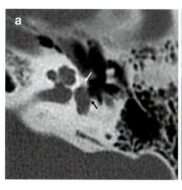 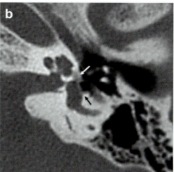 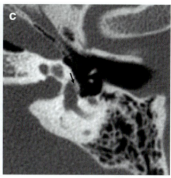

Fig. 2.36 Transversal computed tomography of left ears: (**a**) normal thin aspect of the footplate (*black arrow*), very small prevestibular otospongiotic focus (*white arrow*); (**b**) moderate otosclerotic footplate thickening (*black arrow*) with a large prevestibular focus (*white arrow*); (**c**) obliterating footplate otosclerosis (*black arrow*)

2.6.2.6 The Round Window

The round window is the second opening of the labyrinth to the middle ear. The round window niche is located in the posteroinferior aspect of the promontory in the medial wall of the tympanic cavity. The round window niche is closed by the round window membrane.

The round window niche is never more than 2 mm from the inferior margin of the oval window and is separated from the promontory by the subiculum. The round window niche varies in depth up to approximately 1 mm and is usually triangular in shape, having anterior, posterosuperior and posteroinferior walls [45–50] (Figs. 2.30 and 2.31).

The posterosuperior and posteroinferior walls meet posteriorly leading to the sinus tympani (Fig. 2.30). The anterior and posteroinferior margin of the round window overlies a crest (*crista fenestra*), which projects a mean distance of 0.2 mm; it must be drilled away during cochlear implantation to insure a good exposure and to allow the electrode to pass tangentially along the basal turn of the cochlea [49].

Surgical Application
The ampulla of the posterior semicircular canal is the closest vestibular structure to the round window. The nerve supplying this ampulla, *singular nerve*, lies close to the round window niche. The round window forms a landmark for the position of the singular nerve. The singular canal that contains the nerve lies immediately inferior to the posterior attachment of the round window membrane.

Near the round window, the cochlear aqueduct connects the scala tympani (perilymph) with the subarachnoid space CSF.

Large hypotympanic cells of the hypotympanum border inferiorly the round window niche. These prominent cells must not to be mistaken as the round window niche, especially during cochlear implant surgery.

Clinical Implication
The round window is the second most common site of otosclerosis. Round window involvement varies from mild involvement of the edge to a complete obliteration of the niche. Round window involvement could be diagnosed and staged by HRCT scan with thin cuts and classified from RW1 to RW5 [50] (Fig. 2.37).

Round Window Membrane
The round window membrane lies in the round window niche obscured to a variable degree by a bony overhang, which extends over the membrane anteriorly and superiorly for a distance of up to 1 mm [49, 50]. The round window membrane is placed at a right angle to the plane of the footplate.

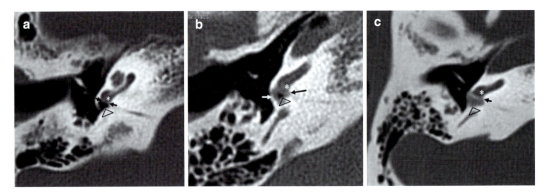

Fig. 2.37 Computed tomography in the transversal plan of right ears showing (**a**) normal round window membrane (*between the small black arrows*), very thin limit between the air filled round window recess (*arrowhead*) and the endolymph in the scala tympani of the basal turn of the cochlea (*) (**b**) otosclerotic foci on the promontory (*white arrow*) and of the round window (*black arrow*), presence of air in round window recess (*arrowhead*), but separated from the scala tympani (*) by the otosclerotic focus: RW3 (**c**) Condensation of the round window membrane (*black arrow*), scala tympani (*), complete obliteration of the round window recess (*arrowhead*): RW4

Clinical Application

The promontory covers completely the round window membrane which is oriented inferiorly and posteriorly. Therefore, in a transcanal approach, it is impossible to see the membrane per se directly. The correct assessment of a diseased round window membrane such as in otosclerosis with its different stages or an invasive tympanosclerosis is only possible with thin-cut computed tomography [50]. In addition a good access to the membrane requires surgical removal of the superior overhang of the niche. Moreover, some strands draped over the RW niche, remnants of embryonic connective tissue, render the RW membrane difficult to be seen (Fig. 2.38).

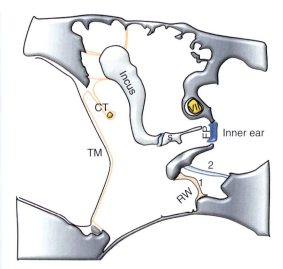

Fig. 2.38 Schematic drawing showing the round window (*RW*) with its false membrane (*1*) and true membrane (*2*). *S* stapes, *TM* tympanic membrane, *FP* footplate, *CT* chorda tympani

The mean horizontal diameter of the round window membrane is 1.35 mm and the vertical diameter 1.79 mm [46–50]. The membrane does not lie at the end of the scala tympani but forms part of its floor. The hook region of the basal turn of the cochlea is a cul-de-sac lying posterior to the round window.

The thickness of the normal human RWM is 60–70 μm [51]. The ultrastructure of the RWM consists of an outer epithelium of low cuboidal cells lining the middle ear, an inner epithelium of squamous cells bordering the inner ear, and a layer of connective tissue between the epithelial layers. The connective tissue layer consists of fibroblasts, collagen, and elastic fibers.

The membrane has several functions [52]: It releases mechanical energy to the labyrinthine fluids, permitting movement of the inner ear fluids associated with the movements of the stapedial footplate; thus, patency of the niche is essential for efficient acoustic transmission; it can serve as an alternative route for sound energy to enter the cochlea.

Clinical Application
Passage through the membrane is possible for small molecules by passive diffusion and for larger molecules probably by endocytosis [53, 54]. The round window membrane acts as the main gateway for local therapy of inner ear diseases. Drugs (such as dexamethasone and gentamicin) or bacterial exotoxins (in case of acute and chronic otitis media) present in the middle ear may pass through the round window membrane to reach the inner ear [55].

References

1. Langman J. Embryologie Médicale. Paris: Masson; 1965. p. 34.
2. Michaels L. An epidermoid formation in the developing middle ear: possible source of cholesteatoma. J Otolaryngol. 1986;15(3):169–74.
3. Michaels L. Origin of congenital cholesteatoma from a normally occurring epidermoid rest in the developing middle ear. Int J Pediatr Otorhinolaryngol. 1988;15(1): 51–65.
4. Paço J, Branco C, Estibeiro H, Oliveira E, Carmo D. The posterosuperior quadrant of the tympanic membrane. Otolaryngol Head Neck Surg. 2009;140(6):884–8.
5. Shrapnell HJ. On the form and structure of the membrane timpani. London Med Gazette. 1832;10: 120–4.
6. Henson Jr OW, Henson MM. The tympanic membrane: highly developed smooth muscle arrays in the annulus fibrosus of mustached bats. J Assoc Res Otolaryngol. 2000;1:25–32.
7. Adad B, Ragson BM, Ackerson L. Relationship of the facial nerve to the tympanic annulus: a direct anatomic examination. Laryngoscope. 1999;109:1189–92.
8. Makino K, Amatsu M. Epithelial migration on the tympanic membrane and external canal. Arch Otorhinolaryngol. 1986;243(1):39–42.
9. Lim DJ. Tympanic membrane: electron microscopic observations, part I: pars tensa. Acta Otolaryngol. 1968; 66:181–98.
10. Lim DJ. Structure and function of the tympanic membrane: a review. Acta Otorhinolaryngol Belg. 1995;49:101–15.
11. Lim DJ. Tympanic membrane: electron microscopic observations, part II: pars fláccida. Acta Otolaryngol. 1968;66:515–32.
12. Sadé J. Retraction pockets and attic cholesteatomas. Acta Otorhinolaryngol Belg. 1980;34:62–84.
13. Spector GJ, Ge XX. Development of the hypotympanum in the human fetus and neonate. Ann Otol Rhinol Laryngol Suppl. 1981;90(6 Pt 2):1–20.
14. Friedmann DR, Eubig J, McGill M, Babb JS, Pramanik BK, Lalwani AK. Development of the jugular bulb: a radiologic study. Otol Neurotol. 2011;32(8):1389–95.
15. Roland Jr JT, Hoffman RA, Miller PJ, Cohen NL. Retrofacial approach to the hypotympanum. Arch Otolaryngol Head Neck Surg. 1995;121(2):233–6.
16. Graham MD. The jugular bulb: its anatomic and clinical considerations in contemporary otology. Laryngoscope. 1977;87(1):105–25.
17. Friedmann DR, Le BT, Pramanik BK, Lalwani AK. Clinical spectrum of patients with erosion of the inner ear by jugular bulb abnormalities. Laryngoscope. 2010;120(2):365–72.
18. Eby TL. Development of the facial recess: implications for cochlear implantation. Laryngoscope. 1996;106 (5 Pt 2 Suppl 80):1–7.
19. Miklós Tóth, Pre- and postnatal changes in the human tympanic cavity, Semmelweis University School of Doctoral Studies for Developmental Biology Ph.D. Thesis, Budapest; 2007.
20. Sanna M, Fois P, Paolo F, Russo A, Falcioni M. Management of meningoencephalic herniation of the temporal bone: personal experience and literature review. Laryngoscope. 2009;119:1579–85.
21. De Carpentier J, Axon PR, Hargreaves SP, Gillespie JE, Ramsden RT. Imaging of temporal bone brain hernias: atypical appearances on magnetic resonance imaging. Clin Otolaryngol. 1999;24:328–34.
22. Toth M, Helling K, Baksa G, Mann W. Localization of congenital tegmen tympani defects. Otol Neurotol. 2007;28:1120–3.
23. Weber PC. Iatrogenic complications from chronic ear surgery. Otolaryngol Clin North Am. 2005;38:711–22.
24. Lang J. Skull base and related structures: atlas of clinical anatomy. 2nd ed. Stuttgart: Schattauer; 2001.
25. Horn KL, Brackman DE, Luxford WM, Shea III JJ. The supratubal recess in cholesteatoma surgery. Ann Otol Rhinol Laryngol. 1986;95:12–5.
26. Schuknecht HF, Gulya AJ. Anatomy of the temporal bone with surgical implications. Philadelphia: Lea & Febiger; 1986. p. 89–90.
27. Makki FM, Amoodi HA, van Wijhe RG, Bance M. Anatomic analysis of the mastoid tegmen: slopes and tegmen shape variances. Otol Neurotol. 2011;32(4): 581–8.
28. Tóth M, Medvegy T, Moser G, Patonay L. Development of the protympanum. Ann Anat. 2006;188(3):267–73.
29. Potter GD, Graham MD. The carotid canal. Radiol Clin North Am. 1974;12:483–9.
30. Grand CM, Louryan S, Bank WO, Balériaux D, Brotchi J, Raybaud C. Agenesis of the internal carotid artery and cavernous sinus hypoplasia with

contralateral cavernous sinus meningioma. Neuroradiology. 1993;35(8):588–90.

31. Savic D, Djeric D. Anatomical variations and relations in the medial wall of the bony portion of the eustachian tube. Acta Otolaryngol. 1985;99(5–6):551–6. doi:10.3109/00016488509182260.

32. PenidoNde O, Borin A, Fukuda Y, Lion CN. Microscopic anatomy of the carotid canal and its relations with cochlea and middle ear. Braz J Otorhinolaryngol. 2005; 71(4):410–4.

33. Hasebe S, Sando I, Orita Y. Proximity of carotid canal wall to tympanic membrane: a human temporal bone study. Laryngoscope. 2003;113(5):802–7.

34. Young RJ, Shatzkes DR, Babb JS, Lalwani AK. The cochlear-carotid interval: anatomic variation and potential clinical implications. AJNR Am J Neuroradiol. 2006;27(7):1486–90.

35. Jahrsdoerfer RA. Embryology of the facial nerve. Am J Otol. 1988;9:423–6.

36. Nager GT, Proctor B. Anatomical variations and anomalies involving the facial canal. Otolaryngol Clin North Am. 1991;24:531–53.

37. Jahrsdoerfer RA. Congenital absence of the oval window. ORL J Otorhinolaryngol Relat Spec. 1977;84: 904–14.

38. Harada T, Black FO, Sand OI, Singleton GT. Temporal bone histopathologic findings in congenital anomalies of the oval window. Otolaryngol Head Neck Surg. 1980;88:275–87.

39. Gerhardt HJ, Otto HD. The intratemporal course of the facial nerve and its influence on the development of the ossicular chain. Acta Otolaryngol. 1981;91: 567–73.

40. Lambert PR. Congenital absence of the oval window. Laryngoscope. 1990;100:37–40.

41. Zeifer B, Sabini P, Sonne J. Congenital absence of the oval window: radiologic diagnosis and associated anomalies. AJNR Am J Neuroradiol. 2000;21(2): 322–7.

42. Cauldwell EW, Anson BJ. Stapes, fissula ante fenestram and associated structures in man. II. From embryos 6.7 to 50 mm in length. Arch Otolaryngol. 1942;36:891–925.

43. Anson BJ, Cauldwell EW, Bast TH. The fissula ante fenestram of the human otic capsule. II. Aberrant

form and contents. Ann Otol Rhinol Laryngol. 1948;57:103–28.

44. Linder TE, Ma F, Huber A. Round window atresia and its effect on sound transmission. Otol Neurotol. 2003;24(2):259–63.

45. Nomura Y. Otological significance of the round window. Adv Otorhinolaryngol. 1984;33:1–162.

46. Su WY, Marion MS, Hinojosa R, Matz GJ. Anatomical measurements of the cochlear aqueduct, round window membrane, round window niche, and facial recess. Laryngoscope. 1982;92(5):483–6.

47. Franz BK, Clark GM, Bloom DM. Surgical anatomy of the round window with special reference to cochlear implantation. J Laryngol Otol. 1987;101(2):97–102.

48. Paprocki A, Biskup B, Kozłowska K, Kuniszyk A, Bien D, Niemczyk K. The topographical anatomy of the round window and related structures for the purpose of cochlear implant surgery. Folia Morphol (Warsz). 2004;63(3):309–12.

49. Li PM, Wang H, Northrop C, Merchant SN, Nadol Jr JB. Anatomy of the round window and hook region of the cochlea with implications for cochlear implantation and other endocochlear surgical procedures. Otol Neurotol. 2007;28(5):641–8.

50. Mansour S, Nicolas K, Ahmad HH. Round window otosclerosis: radiologic classification and clinical correlations. Otol Neurotol. 2011;32(3):384–92.

51. Sahni RS, Paparella MM, Schachern PA, Goycoolea MV, Le CT. Thickness of the human round window membrane in different forms of otitis media. Arch Otolaryngol Head Neck Surg. 1987;113:630–4.

52. Goycoolea MV, Lundman L. Round window membrane. Structure function and permeability: a review. Microsc Res Tech. 1997;36:201–11.

53. Goycoolea MV, Muchow D, Schachern P. Experimental studies on round window structure: function and permeability. Laryngoscope. 1988;98(6 Pt 2 Suppl 44): 1–20.

54. Kim CS, Cho TK, Jinn TH. Permeability of the round window membrane to horseradish peroxidase in experimental otitis media. Otolaryngol Head Neck Surg. 1990;103:918–25.

55. Penha R, Escada P. Round-window anatomical considerations in intratympanic drug therapy for inner-ear diseases. Int Tinnitus J. 2005;11(1):31–3.

Middle Ear Contents

3

Contents

Traditionally, the ossicular chain is considered as the essential content of the middle ear. It is suspended inside the cavity by ligaments and muscles, which will be addressed in their embryological development and their anatomical details in this chapter.

Nowadays, it is admitted in middle ear mechanics that the most important content of the middle ear to assure a normal sound transmission, in addition to the ossicular chain, is gas (air).

The tympanic cavity contains an average of 2 cc of air. The minimal volume of air necessary for a normal function of the middle ear is at least 0.5 cc. Air transmits the sound wave from outside to the tympanic membrane and inside the middle ear, air serves as an insulator. When air of the middle ear is replaced by an effusion, hearing loss will result due to the reduction of pressure difference of the sound wave in between the oval window and the round window with an escape of sound energy to the surrounding bony structures.

Furthermore, the middle ear cavity contains several mucosal folds that divide the middle ear cavity in different compartments and spaces. The folds and their openings define middle ear aeration pathways and play an important role in the evolution of some middle ear pathologies, such as inflammation or cholesteatoma.

S. Mansour et al., *Comprehensive and Clinical Anatomy of the Middle Ear*,
DOI 10.1007/978-3-642-36967-4_3, © Springer-Verlag Berlin Heidelberg 2013

Fig. 3.1 Destination of the first and the second branchial arches. *M* malleus, *I* incus, *S* stapes, *AP* anterior malleal process, (*) double origin of the footplate

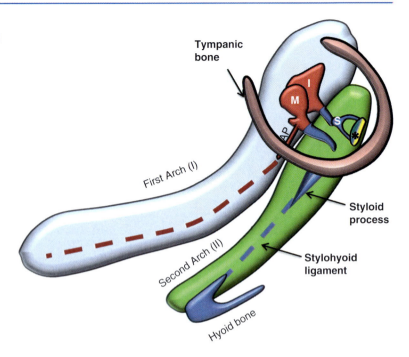

3.1 The Auditory Ossicles

The auditory ossicles are the *malleus*, *incus*, and *stapes*; they are named after the objects they resemble (hammer, anvil, and stirrup). The ossicles are suspended in the middle ear cavity by numerous *suspensory ligaments,* and they are covered by the mucous membrane of the middle ear cavity. The auditory ossicles form the ossicular chain which is responsible for transmission of sound-induced vibrations of the tympanic membrane to the oval window. This system is the cornerstone of middle ear mechanics.

3.1.1 Embryology of the Auditory Ossicles

The ossicles, muscles, and tendons of the middle ear are formed from the mesenchyme of the middle ear and are covered by the epithelial lining of the first pharyngeal pouch [1].

The mesenchyme forming the ossicles is derived from neural crest cells present in the first and second branchial arches. These cells migrate to the branchial arch from the dorsal part of the

developing neural tube during the fourth week of gestation [2].

There is controversy about the contribution of each arch to ossicular formation; there are two main theories regarding this subject:

- *The classical theory:* postulates that the incus and the malleus are derived from Meckel's cartilage of the first branchial arch; the stapes is derived from Reichert's cartilage of the second branchial arch [3–7].
- *The alternative theory*: proposes that the head of the malleus and the body of the incus originate from the first arch, while the handle of the malleus, the long process of the incus, and most of the stapes originate from the second arch (Fig. 3.1) [8–13].

In both theories, the labyrinthine side of the footplate was considered to originate from the mesenchyme of the otic capsule. However, some normal and teratologic observations in the literature support the idea that the stapes could entirely derive from the Reichert's cartilage without any contribution of the otic capsule [14–16].

Ossicular development in the human embryo starts at the fourth week of gestation as an interbranchial mesenchymal bridge connecting

Fig. 3.2 13-mm human embryo. The common blastema of the handle of the malleus and the long crus of the incus (the *two arrows*) crossed by the chorda tympani (*). *TR* tubotympanic recess of the first branchial pouch, *G* first ectodermal groove, *VII* facial nerve in the second branchial arch. Hematoxylin-eosin staining

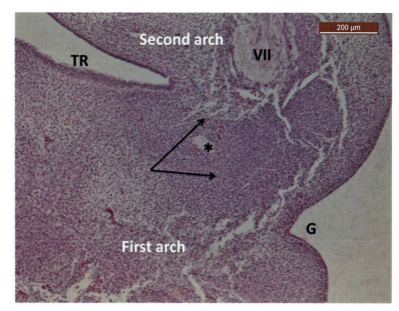

the mesenchyme of the upper part of the first branchial arch and the central part of the second branchial arch. This condensed mesenchyme gives rise to the primordial malleus and incus [12, 17, 18]. This mesenchymal mass is crossed by the chorda tympani that divides it in two parts: the malleal primordium laterally and the incudal primordium medially (Fig. 3.2). This common rudiment keeps connection with the Reichert's cartilage, supporting the "alternative" theory in that all of the stapes blastema derives from the second arch mesenchyme.

During the sixth week, a precartilage forms in the future ossicles. A rapid transformation into true cartilage occurs during the seventh week. By the end of the eighth week, the cartilaginous malleus resembles adult ones. Thereafter, progressive and extensive ossicular growth occurs and, by the 20th week, the ossicles reach adult size and have begun to ossify.

Ossification of the incus takes place slightly earlier than that of the malleus. In the 25th to 26th week, both the incus and malleus are fully ossified with the exception of the distal extremity of the malleus handle. Meanwhile, the pneumatization process of the tympanic cavity extends into the epitympanum and antrum, making the ossicles free only tethered to the tympanic cavity in a mesentery-like fashion.

Clinical Application

Before birth, the ossicles have achieved adult size and shape. The endochondral bone of the ossicles, similar to that of the otic capsule, undergoes only little changes over lifetime of the individual and demonstrates poor reparative capacity in response to fractures.

3.1.1.1 Stapes Development

The stapes, the first ossicle to appear, develops from an independent anlage derived from the cranial end of the cartilage of the second branchial arch (Fig. 3.1). The stapedial anlage connects to the remaining Reichert's cartilage by a formation called the interhyale; the internal part of the interhyale gives rise to the tendon of the stapedial muscle.

The stapedial anlage will be crossed by the stapedial artery during embryonic period, giving the stapes its characteristic ring shape (Fig. 3.3).

Footplate Development

There are two theories regarding the origin of stapedial footplate. Despite the fact that there are several differences between both theories, it is accorded that footplate development is characterized by a progressive replacement of

Fig. 3.3 13-mm human embryo section showing the stapedial (*) rudiment crossed by the stapedial artery (*arrow*). Hematoxylin-eosin staining

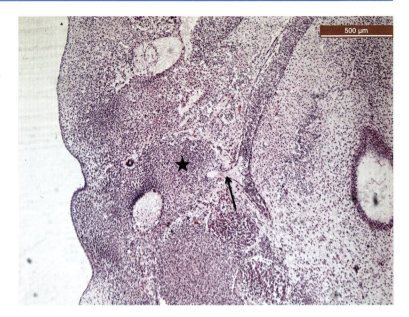

undifferentiated mesenchyme by chondroblasts, and differentiation of the peripheral mesenchyme into the annular ligament around the presumptive footplate, as demonstrated by Jacksoll in the chick embryo [19] (Fig. 3.4).

- *Classical theory of footplate origin*
  The classical theory presumes that the footplate has two origins: the tympanic side derived from the stapedial ring and the vestibular side derived from the lamina stapedialis of the otic capsule [16]. The medial border of the stapedial ring comes in contact with a facing depression in the lateral wall of the otic capsule. This depression, called the *lamina stapedialis*, is the future oval window. The medial border of the stapedial ring fuses with the lamina stapedialis to form the stapedial footplate (Fig. 3.5).
- *Alternative theory of footplate origin*
  According to this theory, the otic capsule is not involved in the formation of the base of the stapes and the entire stapes derives from the stapedial anlage of the Reichert's cartilage [14, 15, 19, 20] (Fig. 3.6).

Annular Ligament

At the beginning, the footplate is attached to the otic capsule by a band of mesenchyme that later transforms into the annular ligament, once the

footplate reaches adult size [19, 20]. The stapediovestibular joint, stapes and the inner ear being decoupled, shows its definitive characteristics at 12th week (Figs. 3.4 and 3.5).

Stapes Ossification

Stapes endochondral ossification starts at the end of the fourth month from a single ossification center present at the center of the footplate. The ossification extends to the two branches and then to the head of the stapes [21].

Clinical Application
Congenital stapes anomalies are sometimes related to an aberrant facial nerve development. During the crucial time period of sixth week, anterior displacement of the second genu region of the facial nerve hinders the normal fusion of the stapedial ring with the lamina stapedialis, resulting in a malformed stapes in conjunction with anomalous facial nerve trajectory.

3.1.1.2 Incus Development

The incus is the second ossicle to appear, but the first to be ossified. The body of the incus derives from the cranial part of the Meckel's

Fig. 3.4 Footplate development in the bird (According to Jaskoll 1980 [19]. (**a**)–(**f**): Successive stages of development of the footplate and related structures. This material is reproduced with permission of John Wiley & Sons, Inc.). Chondroblasts of the otic capsule and stapes are initially separated by undifferentiated mesenchyme. This mesenchyme progressively disappears and becomes present in the "isthmus" (*arrows*) in which will develop the annular ligament. *FP* footplate, *AL* annular ligament, *OC* otic capsule

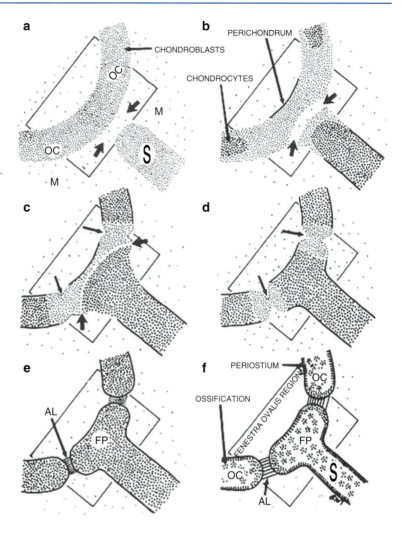

cartilage. The long process of the incus derives from Reichert's cartilage (Figs. 3.1 and 3.7). Endochondral ossification starts at the beginning of the fourth gestational month from the anterior face of the long process and ends at the sixth month reaching adult size.

Clinical Application

Congenital absence of the long process of the incus results in a near-maximal conductive hearing loss [22, 23].

3.1.1.3 Malleus Development

The head of the malleus (Figs. 3.1, 3.7, and 3.8) appears as a mass connected to the cranial end of the Meckel's cartilage. This connection disappears later to be replaced by the anterior process of the malleus and anterior malleal ligament. The anterior process, which can be up to 10 mm in neonates, remains in the adult malleus only as a small prominence. A lack of bony involution can keep the malleus fixed at the petrotympanic fissure [24].

The handle of the malleus has close relationships with the long process of the incus in a blastema originally connected to the Reichert's cartilage.

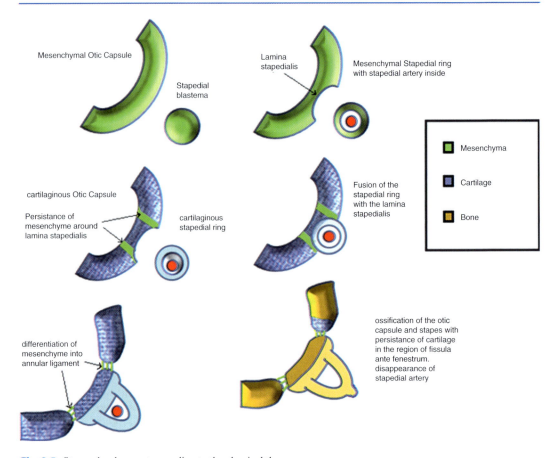

Fig. 3.5 Stapes development according to the classical theory

Failure of resorption of this connection with Reichert's cartilage leads to formation of malleus handle bony bar (see Sect. 3.1.1.4). Later, the handle of malleus becomes inserted in the tympanic membrane rudiment.

This different origin of the head and of the handle of the malleus explains why in aural atresia the head of the malleus is present while the handle is missing. Malleus ossification ends by the sixth month [25].

Congenital Ossicular Malformations

Congenital ossicular malformations could be associated with aural atresia and microtia, or it could be isolated without external ear anomaly as in minor ear atresia. Ossicular anomalies in minor atresia are subdivided into incudomalleal fixation, stapes fixation, and incudostapedial disconnection [26]. Incudomalleal fixations are

the least common, where the malleus head and incus body are usually fused or fixed to the epitympanic walls [27]. Triple ossicular malformations are rare and could be associated with inner ear anomalies [28].

Malleus Congenital Anomalies

The incidence of malleus anomalies is lower than anomalies of the incus or stapes. Hypoplasia or aplasia of the malleus results from a failure of embryogenesis between 7th and 25th week. Given the common pharyngeal arch origin, hypoplasia of the malleus is often associated with hypoplasia of the incus [22].

Epitympanic fixation of the head of malleus is by far the most congenital anomaly of the malleus. This anomaly is related to an incomplete pneumatization of the epi-tympanum during malleus head ossification. Temporal bone exploration in these patients reveals bony bridges between the head of the malleus and the lateral epitympanum in the majority of cases [24, 27] (Fig. 3.9).

Malleus bar is a persistent bony bridge that connects the malleus handle to the posterior tympanic wall [29, 30].

Incus Congenital Anomalies
Hypoplasia or aplasia of the incus typically occurs in conjunction with hypoplasia of the malleus but may occur in isolation. The incus is also susceptible to fixation to the epitympanum (Fig. 3.9). Congenital absence of the long process of the incus might be associated with aplasia of the stapes and of the handle of malleus, supporting the hypothesis of their common origin [22, 23] (Fig. 3.10).

Stapes Congenital Anomalies
Congenital stapes footplate fixation is the most common isolated ossicular anomaly, approximately 40 % of all congenital ossicular malformations. It is thought to result from ossification of the peripheral mesenchyme of the footplate instead of differentiating into the annular ligament [31].

Although aplasia of the stapes is rare, multiple forms of hypoplasia that include small or absent crura and blob-like stapes have been described. In contrast, isolated hyperplasia of the stapes is often an incidental finding that does not require therapy; this anomaly is thought to result from a failure of the resorption and remodeling that occurs during the final stages of stapes development. Several crural anomalies have been described, including thin, absent, fused, and angled crura. The crura may also be replaced with a columella-like

structure. Congenital stapes disorders are often related to aberrant facial nerve development [10, 22, 32].

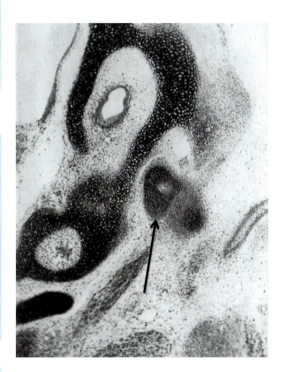

Fig. 3.6 E16 mouse embryo whose mother received a teratogen molecule (methyl triazene) disturbing ossicles formation. A complete stapes develops independently from the otic capsule (*arrow*). In front of the stapes, we observe a narrowing of the otic capsule cartilage. Toluidine blue staining at pH2

3.1.2   Anatomy of the Auditory Ossicles

3.1.2.1 The Malleus
The malleus is shaped like a hammer and is the largest of the three middle ear ossicles. It is 8–9 mm in length and weighs about 20–25 mg. It consists of a head, neck, handle, and two processes arising from below the neck (Fig. 3.11).

The Malleus Head
The malleus head lies in the attic region of the middle ear and is 2.5 by 2 mm in size. On its posteromedial surface, there is an elongated saddle-shaped facet to articulate with the incus. This facet is covered by an articular cartilage.

Fig. 3.7 Sagittal section
of E17 mouse embryo
displaying the cartilaginous
malleus (*M*), incus (*I*),
and stapes (*S*) in close
relationship with the otic
capsule (*O*). The incudomal-
lear joint is just forming (***).
Toluidine blue staining at
pH4

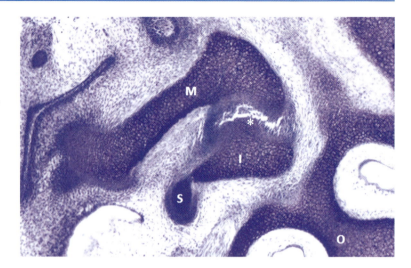

Fig. 3.8 Coronal section of a
19-mm human embryo
revealing the coalescence of
the handle of malleus (*Ha*)
and the head of malleus (*He*).
The handle projects between
the first ectodermal groove
(*G*) and the first endodermal
pouch (*TR*). At this stage, the
ossicles are cartilaginous.
Hematoxylin-eosin staining

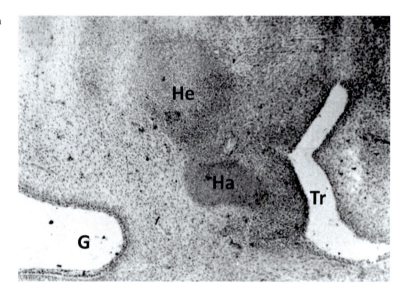

Fig. 3.9 (**a**) Transversal
computed tomography of a
right ear: bony bridge
(*arrow*) between the malleus
head and the tegmen.
(**b**) Transversal computed
tomography of a left ear
with fixation of the incus
on the medial attic wall
(*black arrow*), malleus
head (*white arrow*)

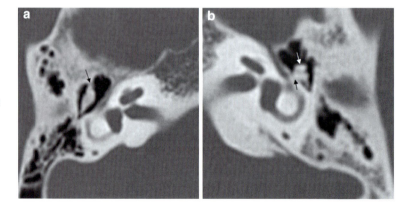

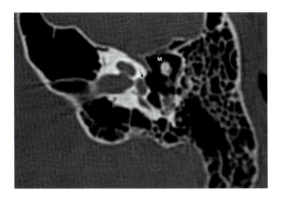

Fig. 3.10 Computed tomography of a left ear with aplasia of stapes suprastructure and the long process of the incus. *M* malleus; stapes footplate (*arrow*)

Malleus Head Fixation: Malleus head fixation is not an uncommon pathology. It may be a congenital anomaly (Fig. 3.9) or acquired anomaly as in tympanosclerosis (Fig. 3.12). Clinically it manifests as a 15–25-dB conductive hearing loss [33].

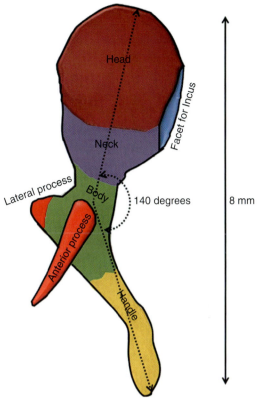

Fig. 3.11 Schematic drawing of the malleus

The Neck

The neck is a narrow and flattened portion. The tendon of the tensor tympani muscle inserts on its medial surface, and the chorda tympani crosses its medial surface above the insertion of this tendon. Its lateral surface forms the medial wall of the Prussak's space.

The Manubrium (The Handle)

The handle forms with the malleus head a superoposteriorly open angle of 135–140°. It runs downwards, medially, and slightly backwards between the mucous and fibrous layers of the tympanic membrane. The inferior end of the handle is flattened and firmly attached to the tympanic membrane as the pars propria splits to envelop it forming the *umbo*.

In surgical procedures, the tympanic membrane can be readily separated from the malleus except at the umbo. At the level of the umbo, the periosteum of the handle continues directly with the fibrous layer. Midway between the lateral process and the umbo, the handle has a gentle medial curvature. At this level the handle is not embedded in the tympanic

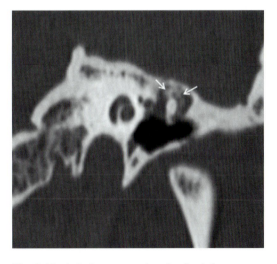

Fig. 3.12 Attical tympanosclerosis of a left ear, computed tomographic coronal reconstruction showing calcifications (tympanosclerosis, *arrows*), surrounding and fixing the malleus to the tegmen

membrane, rather it is linked to the tympanic membrane by a mucosal fold, the *plica mallearis*. A prosthesis clamped to the manubrium in this area may have little or no contact with the pars propria of the normal tympanic membrane and therefore present a very low risk of extrusion (Fig. 3.13).

Malleus Processes

The malleus has two processes located at the union of the neck and the malleus handle.

- *The lateral process*
  The lateral process is a small conical eminence of 1 mm. It protrudes laterally to the side of the tympanic membrane and gives attachment to the anterior and posterior tympano-malleal ligaments.
- The anterior process (*processus gracilis*)
  The anterior process is a 3–5-mm long thin bony spine which extends from the neck of the malleus into the petrotympanic Glaserian fissure. On its medial aspect runs the chorda tympani nerve to enter anteriorly the petrotympanic fissure. It gives origin to the anterior malleal ligament, which also traverses the petrotympanic fissure to reach the angular spine of the sphenoid bone. An extremely long anterior process extending into the petrotympanic fissure may hinder the free movement of the malleus, with little impact on hearing, about 5-dB hearing loss.

Malleus Ligaments (Fig. 3.14)

The malleus is stabilized in place by five ligaments, one articulation, one tendon, and the tympanic membrane. Three of the five ligaments are outside the axis of rotation: they offer only a suspensory function. They are:

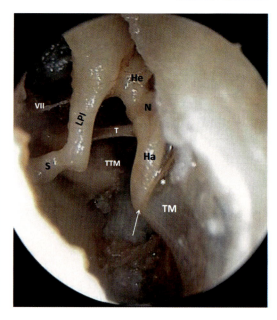

Fig. 3.13 Posterior view of a right middle ear cavity. The inferior end of the handle (*Ha*) is firmly attached to the tympanic membrane (*TM*) forming the umbo (*white arrow*). Relation of the middle part of the handle and the lamina propria of the tympanic membrane (*black arrow*). P*lica mallearis* (*). *LPI* long process of the incus, *S* stapes, *N* neck of the malleus, *He* head of the malleus, *VII* facial nerve, *TTM* tensor tympani muscle, *T* tensor tympani tendon

- *The anterior suspensory ligament (ASL)* lies superior to the anterior malleal ligament and attaches the head of the malleus to the anterior wall of the epitympanum.
- *The lateral suspensory ligament (LSL)* attaches the neck of the malleus to the bony margins of the tympanic notch (the notch of Rivinus) and forms the superior wall of the Prussak's space.
- *The superior suspensory ligament (SSL)* bridges the gap between the head of the malleus and the tegmen of the epitympanum and carries the superior tympanic artery branch of the middle meningeal artery.
  These three ligaments apparently do not interfere with sound transmission because of the small movements of the ossicles at their points of attachment. The suspensory ligaments do not play a role in middle ear mechanics.
- *The anterior malleal ligament (AML)* together with the posterior incudal ligament serves to establish the axis of rotation of the ossicles. The anterior malleal ligament must not be

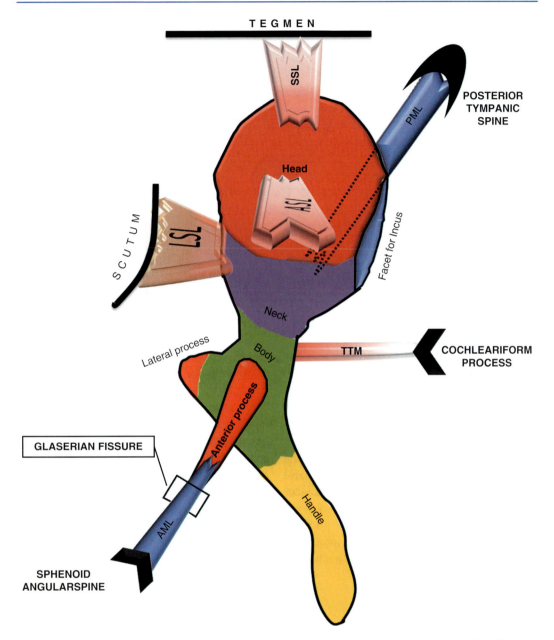

Fig. 3.14 Schema showing malleal ligaments and tensor tympani muscle tendon (*TTM*). *SSL* superior suspensory ligament, *ASL* anterior suspensory ligament, *LSL* lateral suspensory ligament, *AML* anterior malleal ligament, *PML* posterior malleal ligament. The AML and PML in *blue color* represent the axis of rotation of the malleus

confused with the anterior suspensory ligament of the malleus. The anterior malleal ligament extends from the angular spine of the sphenoid bone, passes through the petrotympanic fissure, accompanied by the anterior tympanic artery, and inserts on the neck of the malleus at the base of the anterior process of the malleus.

- *The posterior malleal ligament (PML)* extends from the neck of the malleus to the posterior tympanic spine.

3.1.2.2 The Incus (Fig. 3.15)
The incus measures about 5 by 7 mm and weighs about 30 mg. It has a trapezoidal body, short process, long process, and a rounded *lenticular process*.

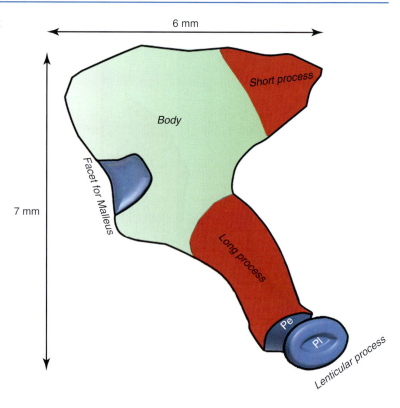

Fig. 3.15 Schematic drawing of the incus. *Pe* lenticular process pedicle, *Pl* lenticular process plate

Body of the Incus

The body of the incus is flat. Its anterior surface houses an elliptical articular surface to receive the head of the malleus. Both body of the incus and the head of the malleus are situated in the attic. Two spines arise from the lower posterior part of the body, the long and short processes. These two processes diverge from each other in a right angle:

Short Process of the Incus

The short process of the incus extends posteriorly from the body as a thick and triangular process; its major axis is horizontal. Its dorsal end lies on the incudal fossa situated in the floor of the aditus ad antrum.

Long Process of the Incus

The long process or vertical process of the incus follows a direction similar to the handle of the malleus but in a more posterior and medial plane. Its caudal end forms a hook at a right angle to end up with the lenticular process. The horizontal,

cross-sectional configuration of the long process of the incus is circular, in contrary to the ovoid shape of the manubrium of the malleus. The mean diameter of the distal extremity of the long process is 0.63 mm [34].

Because of its terminal and poor vascularization, the long process of the incus is highly susceptible to osteitic resorption secondary to several conditions such adhesive otitis media or extremely tightened stapes prosthesis.

Lenticular Process

The lenticular process connects the long process of the incus to the head of the stapes. The lenticular process consists of a narrow *bony pedicle* and a flattened *distal plate*.

The bony pedicle is surrounded by a joint capsule of thick fibers. The mean diameter of the bony pedicle (0.26 mm) is less than half of the mean diameter of the distal long process (0.63 mm) and less than half of the mean diameter of the distal plate (0.71 mm) [34]. The bony pedicle is flexible and plays a role in the piston-like transmission of the incus movement to the stapes, lateral to medial, by the rotation movement of the incus. All other movements are reduced by the bending of this pedicle before reaching the stapes [35].

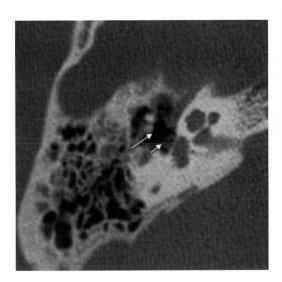

Fig. 3.16 Axial computed tomographic view of a right ear showing a necrosis of the long process secondary to chronic otits media: empty space between the intact stapes (*short arrow*) and the rest of the incus (*long arrow*)

Ligaments of the Incus (Fig. 3.17)

The incus has the least number of ligaments and is therefore more susceptible to traumatic dislocation compared to other ossicles. Two ligaments stabilize the incus in place:

- *The posterior incudal ligament* (*PIL*) secures the short process in the incudal fossa.
- *The superior incudal ligament* (*SIL*) descends from the tegmen to the incus body. It could be reduced to a single mucosal fold only.

3.1.2.3 The Stapes (Fig. 3.18)

The stapes is the smallest bone of the human body; it is 3.25 mm high and 1.4 mm wide with a weight of 3–4 mg [39]. It is situated in an almost horizontal plane between the lenticular process and the oval window and below the facial nerve canal. The stapes consists of a round head, a short neck, anterior and posterior crura, and an oval footplate.

The Head

The head is the most lateral part of the stapes. It is cylindrical or discoid in shape and bears laterally a glenoid cavity, the fovea, which corresponds to the articular surface of the lenticular process. Its medial end is constricted, forming the neck. Its anterior edge is smooth. Its posterior edge presents a small rough surface for the insertion of the stapedial muscle tendon.

The Crura

The stapes presents two unequal crura: the posterior and the anterior crura; the posterior crus is longer, thicker, and more curved than the anterior one. The relative thickness, the curvature, and the excavation of the crura vary among individuals. The area delimited by the concave arches of the crura is the *obturator foramen*, sometimes bridged by a veil of mucous membrane. The two crura could be very close to the walls of the niche of the oval window.

Fig. 3.17 Schematic drawing of incudal ligaments. *SIL* superior incudal ligament, *PIL* posterior incudal ligament

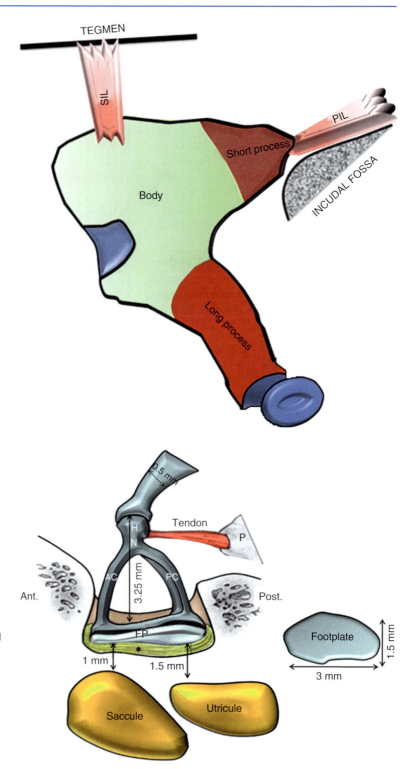

Fig. 3.18 Schematic drawing of stapes in the oval window niche and its relationship with the underlying saccule and utricle. Stapedial tendon in red. (*) annular ligament, *P* pyramidal eminence, *H* head, *N* neck, *AC* anterior crus, *PC* posterior crus, *FP* footplate

The Footplate

The footplate is a thin and oval lamella of bone. Its length is about 3 mm; its width is about 1.5 mm; its thickness is about 0.25 mm [40].

The lateral or tympanic surface of the footplate is covered by mucoperiosteum of the middle ear; it is slightly twisted around its polar axis so that the anterior half looks to the floor of the vestibule and the posterior part looks up to the tegmen. The distance from the long process of the incus to the tympanic surface of the footplate is about 4 mm.

The medial or vestibular surface of the footplate is flat; it is lined by the endosteum of the otic capsule and is in close relation with the saccule and utricle. The saccule is 1 mm deep from the anterior part of the vestibular surface of the footplate, and the utricle is at 1.5 mm deep from its posterior part (Fig. 3.18).

Annular Ligament

The annular ligament of the stapes is a ring of elastic fibers that attaches the cartilaginous margin of the footplate to the border of the oval window. The fibers of the annular ligament fuse with the periosteum and endosteum all around the oval window borders. The ligament is thinner anteriorly than posteriorly and more mobile anteriorly [41]. Because of the differential thickness between its anterior and posterior aspects, the annular ligament works as a hinge-like attachment of the stapes into the oval window. This type of attachment allows a rocking oscillation of the footplate in the oval window, which is the essential movement for the transmission of high-frequency sounds. Low-frequency sound transmission depends on piston-like movements of the stapes that necessitates elasticity of the whole annular ligament.

3.2   Middle Ear Articulations

3.2.1   Embryology of Middle Ear Articulations

3.2.1.1 The Incudostapedial Joint

At the seventh to eighth week of gestation, the outlines of the lenticular process and of the stapes head are separated by a condensed mesenchyme interzone. After the 12th week of gestation, cavitation phenomena begin in this interzone. The different cavitations consolidate then to form the incudosta-pedial joint at the 16th week of gestation.

The primordium of the capsular ligament develops from the surface of the interzone by a condensation of the surrounding mesenchyme which forms a layer that is continued with the perichondrium of the ossicles [42].

3.2.1.2 The Incudomalleal Joint

The incus and malleus, previously one collection of mesenchyme, separate with formation of the incudomalleal joint at eighth to ninth week by the same mechanism as the incudostapedial joint (Fig. 3.7). Failure of this step results in a fused malleus-incus mass that is commonly found in patients with aural atresia.

3.2.2   Anatomy of Middle Ear Articulations

Middle ear articulation surfaces are lined by cartilage. Each articulation has a true capsule originating from the periosteum of the linked bones and lined by a synovial membrane.

3.2.2.1 The Incudomalleal Articulation

The head of the malleus articulates with the body of the incus in a diarthrodial joint in the attic (Fig. 3.19). The joint cavity is incompletely divided into two compartments by a wedge-shaped articular disk or meniscus. The capsule is trilaminar with (1) the synovial membrane lining the cavity, (2) the mucous membrane of the middle ear, and (3) an intervening fibrous layer.

Partial subluxation of the incudomalleal joint, happening during middle ear surgery, usually heals without sequela. Complete luxation will not heal and ossicular reconstruction is recommended.

3.2.2.2 The Incudostapedial Articulation
(Figs. 3.19 and 3.20)

The incudostapedial articulation is a synovial diarthrodial articulation; it joins the convex

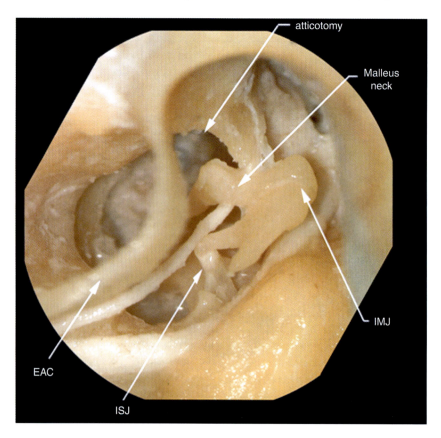

Fig. 3.19 Left middle ear after large mastoidectomy and anterior and posterior tympanotomies, showing both incudo-malleal joint (*IMJ*) and incudostapedial joint (*ISJ*). *EAC* external auditory canal

Fig. 3.20 Computed tomography of the normal appearance of the incudomalleal joint. (**a**) In the transversal view: continuity between the long process of the incus (*arrowhead*) and the head of the stapes (*long arrow*). malleus handle (*short arrow*). (**b**) Coronal reconstruction: continuity between the long process of the incus (*long arrow*) and the head of the stapes (*short arrow*)

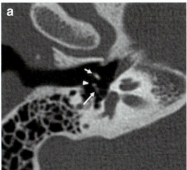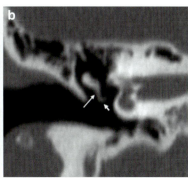

Fig. 3.21 Traumatic lesions of the ossicular chain. (**a**) The long process of the incus (*long arrow*) is displaced anteriorly to the stapes suprastructure (*short arrow*) secondary to traumatic incudostapedial luxation. (**b**) Horizontal temporal bone fracture (*long arrows*) with incudomalleal joint interruption (*short arrow*) and luxation of malleus head anteriorly

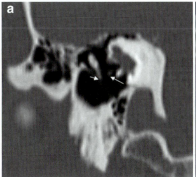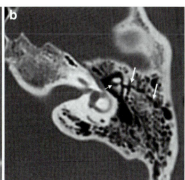

lenticular process of the incus and the concave surface of the head of the stapes. An interarticular cartilage is not usually present. This joint is fragile.

Clinical Implication

Ossicular Chain Trauma (Fig. 3.21)

- Incudostapedial joint separation is the most common ossicular injury in temporal bone trauma.
- Incudomalleal dislocation is the second most common ossicular injury in temporal bone trauma.
- Fracture of the stapes superstructure is the third most frequent ossicular injury in temporal bone trauma.
- Fracture of the malleus is the least common

3.3   Middle Ear Muscles

3.3.1   Embryology of Middle Ear Muscles

The embryological origin of middle ear muscles follows the same patterns as the other muscles in the craniofacial area [43]. They develop from the paraxial mesoderm (mesenchyme) that migrates into the branchial arches.

3.3.1.1 Tensor Tympani Muscle

The tensor tympani muscle develops from the mesoderm of the first branchial arch. It is innervated by a branch from the trigeminal nerve, the nerve of the first branchial arch.

3.3.1.2 Stapedial Muscle

The stapedial muscle starts to develop, at the ninth week, as a condensation of blastema cells in the mesenchyme of the interhyale (which connects the stapedial anlage to the second branchial arch) close to the facial nerve. The internal segment of the interhyale gives rise to the tendon of the stapedial muscle. Moreover, the interhyale contributes to the development of the facial nerve canal, as well as the pyramidal eminence [44] (see Fig. 2.14). The bone of the pyramidal eminence housing the muscle derives from the precartilaginous cells of the second branchial arch [45].

3.3.2 Anatomy of the Middle Ear Muscles

3.3.2.1 The Tensor Tympani Muscle (TTM)

The TTM is fusiform in shape and is around 20 mm in length. The intratympanic portion of this muscle is 2.5 mm long. It arises from the cartilage of the Eustachian tube, from the walls of its enveloping bony semicanal, and from the adjacent portion of the greater wing of the sphenoid bone (Fig. 3.22). The fibers converge to form a central fibrous core which, proceeding posteriorly, forms the tendon of the muscle. The most medial fibers of the tendon attach to the cochleariform process, at which point the main body of the tendon turns laterally into the cavity to attach to the medial surface of the junction of the neck and the manubrium of the malleus (Fig. 3.23). It is innervated by the trigeminal nerve, via the nerve to the medial pterygoid muscle.

The function of the TTM is to draw the manubrium medially, thus tensing the tympanic membrane and damping the movements of the ossicular chain [46, 47].

In normal conditions, the pull of the TTM is opposed by the elasticity of the pars tensa of the tympanic membrane. In a long-standing large perforation of the tympanic membrane, the unopposed pull of the TTM causes a medial displacement of the inferior end of the manubrium (malleus handle medialization).

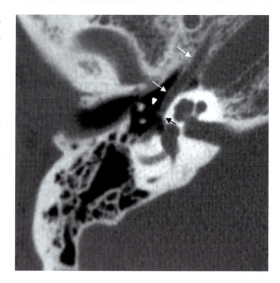

Fig. 3.22 Transversal computed tomography of a right ear, showing the tensor tympani muscle in its bony semicanal (*white arrows*), reaching the cochleariform process (*black arrow*), where its tendon (*white arrowhead*) turns laterally to insert on the neck of the malleus

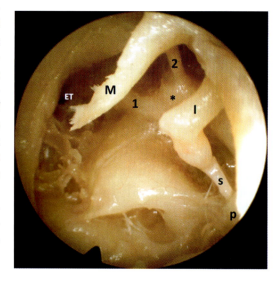

Fig. 3.23 Endoscopic view of a left middle ear showing the stapedial tendon (*s*) rising from the pyramidal process (*p*), the tensor tympani muscle (*1*) turning around the cochleariform process (*) to give the tensor tympani tendon (*2*) that inserts on the neck of malleus (*M*); *I* incus, *ET* Eustachian tube

3.3.2.2 Stapedial Muscle

The stapedial muscle is the smallest skeletal muscle in the body measuring only 1 mm. It lies in a bony cavity in the posterior wall of the tympanic cavity to emerge from the pyramidal eminence. The fibers of this muscle converge into a tendon which variably attaches to the head and/or posterior crus of the stapes (Fig. 3.23) [46, 47].

The stapedial muscle is innervated by the stapedial branch of the facial nerve. Its contraction provokes a tilting of the stapes by moving the anterior border of the footplate laterally and the posterior border medially. This tilting of the stapes stretches the annular ligament, thus fixing the footplate and damping its movements. It protects the inner ear from damage caused by loud noise. Lack of action of this muscle from nerve section or facial nerve palsy induces hyperacusis [46, 47].

> **Surgical Application**
> During microsurgical dissection around the stapes, for instance, a removal of the cholesteatoma matrix from the stapes, it is advisable to work parallel to the plane of the stapedial tendon, from posterior to anterior, so that the tendon prevents luxation of the stapes.

3.4   Middle Ear Nerves

The middle ear receives and transmits branches from the facial nerve, the glossopharyngeal nerve, and the sympathetic carotid plexus. The branches of the glossopharyngeal nerve and sympathetic carotid plexus contribute to the formation of an important middle ear neural plexus, the tympanic plexus.

3.4.1   Facial Nerve Branches

One branch of the facial nerve, the chorda tympani, passes through the middle ear cavity in its route to the infratemporal fossa. This is a sensory and secretory-motor branch of the facial nerve. It enters the middle ear cavity through the *iter chordae posterior*. It runs across the medial surface of the tympanic membrane lateral to the long

process of the incus and passes medial to the upper portion of the handle of the malleus above the tendon of the TTM. It leaves the middle ear through the canal of Huguier placed within the petrotympanic fissure. It joins the lingual branch of the mandibular nerve in the infratemporal fossa (see Sect. 6.2.3.7).

3.4.2   Tympanic Plexus

The tympanic plexus consists of a network of nerves lodged in small grooves on the cochlear promontory of the medial wall of the middle ear. It is formed by the tympanic nerve and two or three filaments from the carotid plexus.

The tympanic (Jacobson's) nerve, carrying parasympathetic fiber, originates from the inferior ganglion of the glossopharyngeal nerve. After entering the tympanic cavity through the medial hypotympanic fissure, it branches repeatedly within shallow bony channels overlying the promontory to form the tympanic plexus.

Two or three filaments, the caroticotympanic nerves, coming from the carotid plexus and carrying sympathetic fibers join the tympanic plexus on the promontory (Fig. 3.24).

The tympanic plexus gives off:
- The lesser petrosal nerve
- Branches to the tympanic cavity mucosa

3.4.2.1 The Lesser Superficial Petrosal Nerve

The lesser superficial petrosal nerve originates from the tympanic plexus at the level of the cochleariform process and leaves the middle ear through a small canal below the tensor tympani muscle (Fig. 3.24). It passes through the temporal bone to emerge on the floor of the middle cranial fossa lateral to the greater superficial petrosal nerve. It exits the middle cranial fossa through the foramen ovale together with the mandibular nerve to join the otic ganglion in the infratemporal fossa. From there, it passes in the auriculotemporal nerve to reach the parotid gland.

The lesser petrosal nerve carries preganglionic parasympathetic fibers of the glossopharyngeal

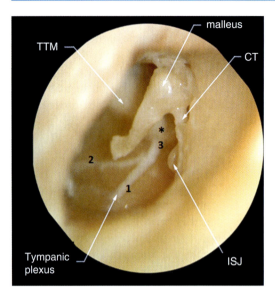

Fig. 3.24 Endoscopic view of a left middle ear showing the Jacobson nerve (*1*), the caroticotympanic nerve (*2*), and the lesser petrosal superficial nerve (*3*) passing outside the middle ear below the cochleariform process (***). *ISJ* incudostapedial joint, *CT* chorda tympani, *TTM* tensor tympani muscle

nerve (IX) to the parotid gland via the otic ganglion. After synapsing in the otic ganglion, postganglionic fibers supply secretory fibers to the parotid gland by the way of the auriculotemporal nerve.

Clinical Application

Tympanic paragangliomas are mostly small-sized tumors originating from the tympanic plexus of the middle ear.

Clinically, these tumors are symptomatic as pulsatile tinnitus and conductive hearing loss. Tympanic paragangliomas are diagnosed by careful otoscopic examination; they appear as a reddish retrotympanic mass behind a translucent tympanic membrane.

Frequently, it is impossible to visualize the entire tumor clinically; thus, computed tomography (CT) or magnetic resonance imaging (MRI) scans are diagnostic (Fig. 3.25).

3.5 Middle Ear Vessels

3.5.1 Embryology of Middle Ear Vessels (Fig. 3.26)

During the 4th week of gestation, the first and second aortic arches begin to involute and they leave behind the mandibular and hyoid arteries, respectively. At the same time the third arch artery becomes the internal carotid artery.

During the 4th to 5th week of gestation, the ventral pharyngeal artery arises from the aortic sac. This artery supplies the bulk of the first two branchial bars and subsequently is involved in the formation of the stapedial and external carotid arteries.

During the 6th week, the stapedial artery arises as a small offshoot of the hyoid artery near its origin from the internal carotid artery. It extends cranially and passes through the stapes blastema to enter the mandibular bar (Fig. 3.3). The stapedial artery divides into two arteries: the maxillomandibular artery and the supraorbital artery (which supplies the primitive orbit). The maxillomandibular division of the stapedial artery joins the distal part of the ventral pharyngeal artery, the future external carotid artery [48].

Over the 7th week, the two major divisions of the stapedial artery are annexed by the internal maxillary artery (from the external carotid artery) and the ophthalmic artery, respectively. The trunk of the maxillomandibular division becomes the stem of the middle meningeal artery. As the stapedial artery withers proximal to the stapes, its more distal stem becomes the superior tympanic branch of the adult middle meningeal artery. The hyoid artery, which gave rise to the stapedial artery, involutes to become a caroticotympanic branch of the internal carotid artery [48].

Persistent Stapedial Artery

Persistent stapedial artery is a rare vascular anomaly of the middle ear. The reported prevalence is of 0.5 % in cadaveric studies [49] and less than the 0.02–0.05 % in

Fig. 3.25 (**a**) Transversal computed tomography with an image of condensation (*arrow*) filling the hypotympanum and covering the inferior half of the promontory.
(**b**) After i.v. injection of iodine contrast, this lesion shows the same contrast uptake (*white arrow*) as the sigmoid sinus (*long black arrow*) and the internal carotid artery (*short black arrow*), confirming a hypervascular lesion

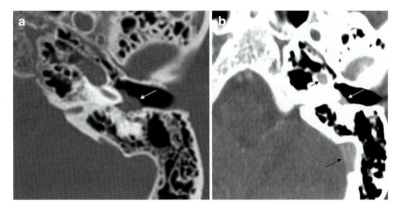

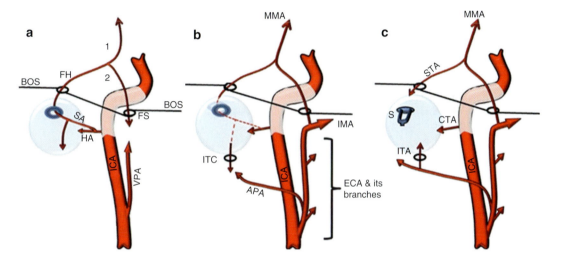

Fig. 3.26 Schema illustrating normal development of middle ear vessels. (**a**) Approximately 6 weeks. (**b**) Approximately 8 weeks. (**c**) Adult configuration. *BOS* base of skull, *FH* facial hiatus, *SA* stapedial artery; blue disk: otic capsule; *HA* hyoid artery, *ICA* internal carotid artery, *FS* foramen spinosum, *VPA* ventral pharyngeal artery, *1* supraorbital artery, *2* maxillomandibular artery, *APA* ascending pharyngeal artery, *ITC* inferior tympanic canaliculus, *MMA* middle meningeal artery, *IMA* internal maxillary artery, *ECA* external carotid artery, *ITA* inferior tympanic artery, *CTA* caroticotympanic artery, *STA* superior tympanic artery, *S* stapes

surgical series [50, 51]. Usually, it is asymptomatic; sometimes, it may cause pulsatile tinnitus and hearing loss [52].

Normally, the stapedial artery atrophies by 3 months of fetal development; however, in very rare cases it may persist as a 1.5- to 2.0-mm branch of the petrous internal carotid artery [52].

A persistent stapedial artery arises from the petrous part of the internal carotid artery, enters the hypotympanum through the medial hypotympanic fissure, crosses the cochlear promontory, and passes through the obturator foramen of the stapes. It enters the Fallopian canal behind the cochleariform process and travels anteriorly with the greater superficial petrosal nerve to enter the middle cranial fossa through the facial hiatus where it ends up as the middle meningeal artery. In case of persistent stapedial artery, the foramen spinosum will be absent [53] (Fig. 3.27).

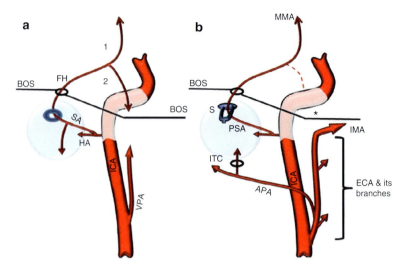

Fig. 3.27 Schema illustrating the development of persistent stapedial artery (PSA). (**a**) Embryonic phase: failure of development of foramen spinosum (*) and communication between maxillomandibular branch (*2*) of stapedial artery (*SA*) and ventral pharyngeal artery (*VPA*). (**b**) Adult configuration of persistent stapedial artery. *BOS* base of skull, *FH* facial hiatus, *SA* stapedial artery, *HA* hyoid artery, *ICA* internal carotid artery, *APA* ascending pharyngeal artery, *ITC* inferior tympanic canaliculus, *MMA* middle meningeal artery, *IMA* internal maxillary artery, *ECA* external carotid artery, *S* stapes

Aberrant Internal Carotid Artery

An aberrant internal carotid artery (ICA) is a variant of the ICA that passes through the middle ear; it appears as a white mass in the anteroinferior quadrant of the middle ear. Otologists should be aware of the possibility of an aberrant ICA when the patient presents with a retrotympanic mass. If mistaken for a tumor and biopsied, the results can be disastrous. Radiological investigation is required to make the differential diagnosis. A temporal bone CT scan in patients with carotid agenesis shows the complete absence of carotid bony canal (see Sect. 2.4.1.1).

The most accepted theory of the etiology of an aberrant internal carotid artery is the agenesis of the vertical internal carotid artery with compensatory vascular communication branches of the developing external carotid artery system. The ascending pharyngeal artery gives rise to the inferior tympanic artery, which is the aberrant internal carotid artery; it then enters the middle ear through the inferior tympanic canaliculus and after passing through the middle ear, it joins the horizontal petrous carotid artery anteriorly (Fig. 3.28).

The presenting signs and symptoms of an aberrant internal carotid artery include pulsatile tinnitus, otalgia, aural fullness, vertigo, and hearing loss [53, 54].

3.5.2 Anatomy of Middle Ear Vessels
(Fig. 3.29)

The blood supply of the middle ear and mastoid cavity originates from the internal and external carotid arteries. We recognize the following important feeding arteries of the middle ear:

3.5.2.1 The Anterior Tympanic Artery
The anterior tympanic artery is a terminal branch of the internal maxillary artery. It gives rise to an important branch, the ossicular branch, which provides the main blood supply for the malleus

Fig. 3.28 Schema illustrating the development of aberrant internal carotid artery. (**a**) Embryonic phase, failure of development of vertical part of internal carotid artery (*ICA*). (**b**) Adult configuration of aberrant carotid artery. Notice the absence of development of the carotid canal. *BOS* base of skull, *ICA* internal carotid artery, *APA* ascending pharyngeal artery, *ITC* inferior tympanic canaliculus, *MMA* middle meningeal artery, *IMA* internal maxillary artery, *ECA* external carotid artery, *ITA* inferior tympanic artery

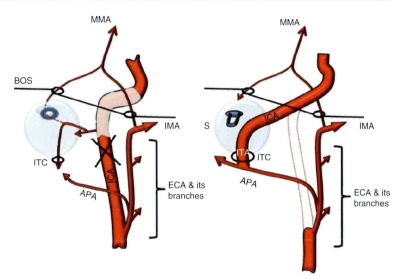

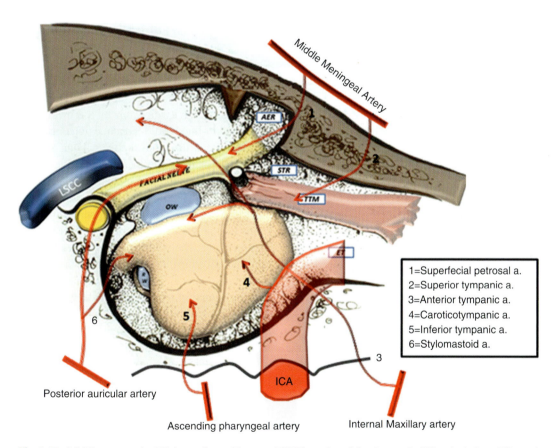

1=Superfecial petrosal a.
2=Superior tympanic a.
3=Anterior tympanic a.
4=Caroticotympanic a.
5=Inferior tympanic a.
6=Stylomastoid a.

Fig. 3.29 Middle ear vessels. *ICA* internal carotid artery, *LSCC* lateral semicircular canal, *OW* oval window, *RW* round window, *AER* anterior epitympanic recess, *STR* supratubal recess, *TTM* tensor tympani muscle, *ET* Eustachian tube

and incus. The anterior tympanic artery also gives rise to branches that supply the bone and mucosa of the superior and lateral walls of the epitympanic cavity.

3.5.2.2 The Posterior Auricular Artery

The posterior auricular artery is another branch of the internal maxillary artery which provides two branches to the vascular ring of the tympanic membrane. A posterior branch supplies most of the tympanic membrane, whereas the anterior branch supplies a lesser portion of the anterior and inferior region.

3.5.2.3 Branches of the Middle Meningeal Artery

The Superficial Petrosal Artery

The superior petrosal artery enters the middle ear through the facial hiatus; it enters the Fallopian canal and provides blood supply to the geniculate ganglion and the tympanomastoid segment of the facial nerve. Also it provides vascularization of the incudostapedial joint and posterior part of stapes by giving rise to the superior and inferior arteries of the stapedial tendon and posterior crural artery.

The Superior Tympanic Artery

The superior tympanic artery enters the middle ear adjacent to the lesser petrosal nerve. The artery supplies the tensor tympani and a portion of the epitympanic space. It also forms an anastomotic plexus with the inferior tympanic artery, giving rise to the anterior stapedial artery and the anterior crural artery.

3.5.2.4 The Caroticotympanic Arteries

The caroticotympanic arteries are branches of the internal carotid artery that pass through the bony wall of the carotid canal to enter the middle ear cleft and eventually anastomose with branches of the inferior tympanic artery.

3.5.2.5 The Inferior Tympanic Artery

The inferior tympanic artery is a branch of the ascending pharyngeal artery; it enters the middle ear cleft with the tympanic (Jacobson's) nerve. This artery, along with the caroticotympanic arteries, provides the major blood supply to the mucosa of the promontory and the lower tympanic cavity (hypotympanum).

3.6 Middle Ear Mucosal Folds

In this section a detailed description of the mucosal folds of the middle ear will be presented in order to clarify their anatomical organization. A good understanding of the anatomy of these folds and their relationships inside the middle ear cavity is fundamental in the learning process of functional middle ear surgery. These folds delimit different compartments, spaces, and recesses, which will be described in detail in Chap. 4.

3.6.1 Mucosal Folds Development

Between the third and seventh fetal months, the mesenchymal tissue of the middle ear cleft is gradually absorbed. At the same time, the primitive tympanic cavity develops by a growth of an endothelium-lined fluid pouch extending from the Eustachian tube into the cleft. Four primary sacci bud out to define the different middle ear spaces. They are the saccus anticus, the saccus medius, the saccus superior, and the saccus posticus [55]. These sacci or pouches start to enlarge in the middle ear cleft to replace the preexisting mesenchyme. The walls of the pouches become the mucosal lining of middle ear cavity. At the plane of contact between two neighboring pouches, mucosal folds are formed. Between the mucosal layers of the folds, there are remnants of the mesenchyme that will transform into ligaments and blood vessels supplying the "viscera" of the tympanic cavity.

3.6.2 Mucosal Folds Anatomy

Middle ear mucosal folds pass from the walls of the middle ear to its contents and carry ligaments and blood vessels to the ossicles. Despite the fact that these folds may orient the progress of middle ear pathologies, they are not true barriers against their extension (Figs. 3.30, 3.31, and 3.32).

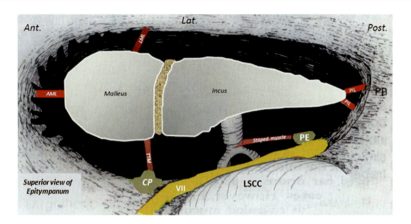

Fig. 3.30 Superior view of a right middle ear, showing middle ear ossicles and their ligaments after removal of all mucosal folds. *AML* anterior malleal ligament, *LML* lateral malleal ligament, *PIL* posterior incudal ligament, *TTM* tensor tympani muscle tendon, *CP* cochleariform process, *PE* pyramidal eminence, *LSCC* lateral semicircular canal, *PB* petrous bone. (Reproduced from Tos [75, fig. 83].With permission from Thieme publishers)

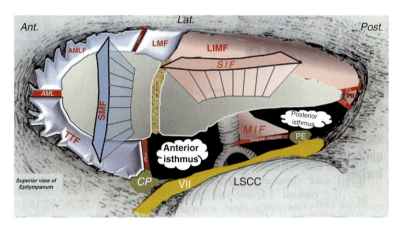

Fig. 3.31 Superior view of a right middle ear showing middle ear ossicles, ligaments, and mucosal folds. *AML* anterior malleal ligament, *LML* lateral malleal ligament, *PIL* posterior incudal ligament, *TTM* tensor tympani muscle tendon, *CP* cochleariform process, *PE* pyramidal eminence, *LSCC* lateral semicircular canal, *TTF* tensor tympani fold, *AMLF* anterior malleal ligamental fold, *LMF* lateral malleal fold, *SMF* superior malleal fold, *MIF* medial incudal fold, *LIMF* lateral incudomalleal fold, *SIF* superior incudal fold, *PIF* posterior incudal fold

There are two different types of mucosal folds: composite folds and duplicate folds.

The composite folds, like the anterior malleal ligamental fold, the lateral malleal ligamental fold, and the posterior incudal fold, have an essential common feature: a combination of a ligament and lining mucosa, with a varying degree of mucosal extension over the ligamental limits and ending with free edges. They are formed when the expanding air sacs meet the preexisting ligament and cover it with mucosal membrane.

The duplicate folds, like the tensor tympani fold and lateral incudomalleal fold, are thin mucosal structures arising from the fusion of two expanding air sac walls in the absence of any interposing structure. Their positions change because the extent of the expansion of each air sac varies in different individuals [56, 57].

3.6.2.1 The Posterior Tympano-Malleal Fold

The posterior tympano-malleal fold, a ligamental fold, inserts on the posterior portion of the neck of the malleus. It involves the upper portion of the handle of the malleus and merges superiorly with the downturn of the anterior portion of the lateral

Fig. 3.32 Posterolateral view of a right middle ear showing middle ear ossicles and mucosal folds. *SMF* superior malleal fold, *SIF* superior incudal fold, *LMF* lateral malleal fold, *AMLF* anterior malleal ligamental fold, *MIF* medial incudal fold, *PIL* posterior incudal ligament, *M* malleus, *LP* lateral process of the malleus. The dotted arrow represents the ventilation tract of the Prussak's space

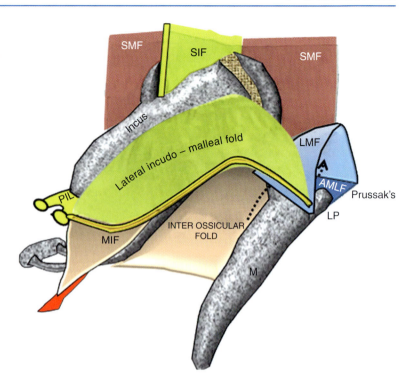

incudomalleal fold. It inserts posteriorly on the posterior tympanic spine and represents the medial wall of the posterior pouch of von Tröltsch. Its medial edge envelops the posterior portion of the chorda tympani [58] (Fig. 3.33).

3.6.2.2 The Anterior Tympano-Malleal Fold

The anterior tympano-malleal fold arises from the anterior portion of the neck of the malleus and inserts anteriorly on the anterior tympanic spine. It forms the medial wall of the anterior pouch of von Tröltsch [58] (Fig. 3.33).

3.6.2.3 The Anterior Malleal Ligamental Fold

The anterior malleal ligamental fold was described by von Tröltsch in 1856. It is part of the tympanic diaphragm. It originates from the neck of the malleus and extends to the anterior attic bony wall. It is reflected from the lateral wall of the middle ear over the anterior process and ligament of the malleus and the anterior part of the chorda tympani.

Its low posterior part is broad and represents the anterior limit of Prussak's space [58] (Fig. 3.34).

3.6.2.4 The Lateral Malleal Ligament Fold

The lateral malleal ligament fold is a thick fold; it is first described by Helmholtz in 1868 [59]. This fold starts from the middle portion of the neck of the malleus to develop a fanlike spread before attaching to the attic outer wall; posteriorly, it is confluent with the anterior descending portion of the lateral incudomalleal fold (Fig. 3.35).

This fold is usually complete; it represents the roof of the Prussak's space and the floor of the lateral malleal space. It is considered to be strong to prevent progression of pars flaccida retraction pockets [60].

Defects in this fold, usually in its thin posterior membranous part, are observed in 7 %. In such cases, the defect provides a direct small communication between the upper and lower epitympanic units [56, 57] (see Sect. 4.5).

3.6.2.5 The Superior Malleal Fold

The superior malleal fold extends between the superior surface of the malleus head and the

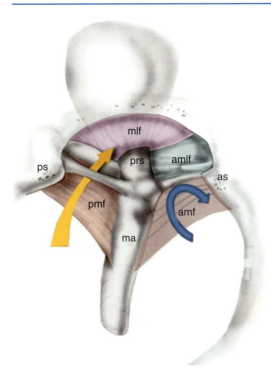

Fig. 3.33 Lateral view of a right middle ear after removal of the tympanic membrane, showing the anterior (*amf*) and the posterior (*pmf*) malleal folds. *as* anterior tympanic spine, *ps* posterior tympanic spine. The *yellow arrow* represents the route of ventilation of the Prussak's space (*prs*). *Blue arrow* represents the complete closure of the Prussak's space floor anteriorly, *mlf* lateral malleal fold, *amlf* anterior malleal ligamental fold, *ma* manubrium. (Reproduced with modification from Marchioni [76, figure 1]. With kind permission from Springer Science and Business Media, Springer and the original publisher)

tegmen in a transversal plane. It contains the superior malleal ligament and divides the attic into anterior and posterior parts (Figs. 3.31 and 3.32).

3.6.2.6 The Lateral Incudomalleal Fold

The lateral incudomalleal fold is a part of the tympanic diaphragm. It lies superiorly in relation to the lateral malleal ligamental fold and separates the upper lateral attic space from the lower lateral attic space. The level of this fold is about 1 mm higher than the roof of the Prussak's space [59]. This fold presents a defect in its anterior portion in about 20 % of cases [57].

The lateral incudomalleal fold has a posterior and a lateral extension: posteriorly, it presents a horizontal extension to insert medially onto the body of the incus and the incudomalleal joint. Laterally, it inserts onto the medial surface of the bony wall of the scutum.

The anterior portion of this fold bends inferiorly towards the neck of the malleus and merges with the posterior portion of the lateral malleal ligament fold, representing the posterior limit of the lateral malleal space (Figs. 3.32 and 3.36).

3.6.2.7 The Medial Incudal Fold

The medial incudal fold is located between the long process of the incus and the tendon of the stapedial muscle as far as the pyramidal eminence (Fig. 3.36).

Fig. 3.34 Superior view of a right middle ear showing the anterior malleal ligamental fold (*AMLF*). *AML* anterior malleal ligament, *LML* lateral malleal ligament, *PIL* posterior incudal ligament, *TTM* tensor tympani muscle tendon, *CP* cochleariform process, *PE* pyramidal eminence, *LSCC* lateral semicircular canal, *PB* petrous bone

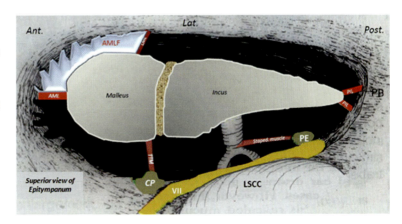

Fig. 3.35 Superior view of a right middle ear showing the lateral malleal fold (*LMF*). *AML* anterior malleal ligament, *LML* lateral malleal ligament, *PIL* posterior incudal ligament, *TTM* tensor tympani muscle tendon, *CP* cochleariform process, *PE* pyramidal eminence, *LSCC* lateral semicircular canal, *PB* petrous bone

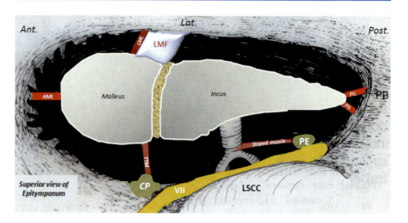

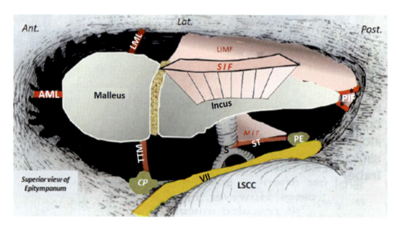

Fig. 3.36 Superior view of the right middle ear, showing the superior incudal fold (SIF), the medial incudal fold (*MIF*), the lateral incudomalleal fold (*LIMF*), and the posterior incudal fold (*PIF*). *TTM* tensor tympani muscle, *ST* stapedial tendon, *AML* anterior malleal ligament, *LML* lateral malleal ligament, *CP* cochleariform process, *VII* facial nerve, * posterior incudal ligament, *S* stapes, *PE* pyramidal eminence, *LSCC* lateral semicircular canal

3.6.2.8 The Superior Incudal Fold (SIF)

The superior incudal fold extends like the superior incudal ligament from the superior surface of the incudal body to the tegmen. It divides the posterior attic into lateral and medial attic (Fig. 3.36).

3.6.2.9 Posterior Incudal Fold

The posterior incudal fold is the fold that runs between the fibers of the posterior incudal ligament (Fig. 3.36).

3.6.2.10 The Tensor Tympani Fold (TTF)

The TTF is a part of the tympanic diaphragm. It arises posteriorly from the tensor tympani tendon, about 1.5 mm lower than the roof of Prussak's space [61]. It runs anteriorly towards the anterior wall of the attic inserting into a transverse crest: the

supratubal ridge. Medially it inserts on the bony canal of the TTM and laterally it inserts on the anterior malleal ligament. The lateral part of the tensor fold keeps a close relationship with the most anterior portion of chorda tympani (Fig. 3.37). It separates the anterior epitympanic recess superiorly from the supratubal recess inferiorly.

Embryologically, the TTF results from the fusion of the saccus anticus and the anterior saccule of the saccus medius. The inclination angle of the TTF varies between 80° and 120° depending on the variable growth of each saccus [62, 63]. The size of the supratubal recess and the anterior epitympanic recess is dependent on the vertical orientation of the TTF. The more vertical the TTF is, the wider is the supratubal recess [61] (Fig. 3.38). A horizontal TTF results in a very small or even inexistent supratubal recess [62] (Fig. 3.38).

Fig. 3.37 Superior view of a right middle ear showing the tensor tympani fold (*TTF*) that inserts posteriorly on the tensor tympani muscle tendon (*TTM*), laterally on the anterior malleal ligament (*AML*), and anteriorly on the anterior attic wall. *LML* lateral malleal ligament, *PIL* posterior incudal ligament, *CP* cochleariform process, *PE* pyramidal eminence, *LSCC* lateral semicircular canal, *PB* petrous bone

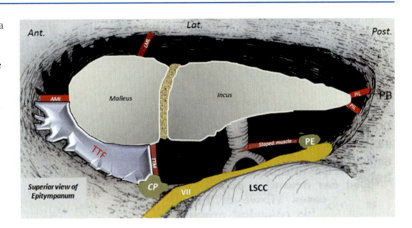

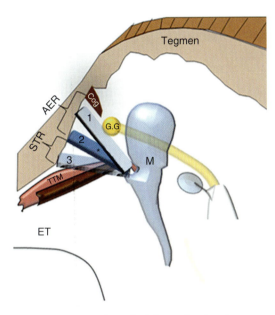

Fig. 3.38 Lateral view of a left ear showing the tensor tympani fold (***) with its variable anterior insertion (*1* high insertion, *2* intermediate insertion, *3* low insertion). The variable insertion of the TTF determines the volume of the anterior epitympanic recess (*AER*) which lies above the TTF and the supratubal recess (*STR*) which lies below the TTF. *TTM* tensor tympani muscle, *M* malleus, *GG* geniculate ganglion

The peripheral portion of the TTF is thick while the central portion is thin and transparent. In some ears, the fold is complete leading to a total separation between the anterior epitympanum and protympanum. In the majority of ears, the TTF is incomplete; this allows a direct communication from the Eustachian tube and supratubal recess to the anterior epitympanic recess and then to the posterior attic (Fig. 3.39).

In such cases the direct aeration of the epitympanum prevents the development of attic dysventilation [63].

3.6.3   The Tympanic Diaphragm

Chatellier and Lemoine introduced the concept of the "epitympanic diaphragm" in 1946 [64], upon which the modern theories of tympanic ventilation have been developed. The authors described how the diaphragm was made up of various structures and membranous ligament that form together with the malleus and the incus the floor of the epitympanic compartment.

Palva et al. revised Chatellier's concept of the epitympanic diaphragm and added two other important folds: the TTF and the lateral incudomalleal fold [65, 66]. According to them, the complete tympanic diaphragm is made up of the three malleal ligamental folds (anterior, lateral, and posterior), the posterior incudal fold, the TTF, the lateral incudomalleal fold, and the incus and the malleus [61, 67] (Fig. 3.40).

The tympanic diaphragm is not fully horizontal because its components are on different levels. It separates the upper unit of the attic superiorly from the mesotympanum and the lower unit of the attic, the Prussak's space, inferiorly. The lateral malleal fold separates Prussak's space from the upper unit of the epitympanum; this is why we call the Prussak's space the lower unit of the attic [61] (see Sect. 4.5).

Fig. 3.39 Superior view of a right middle ear showing incomplete tensor tympani fold (*TTF*). *AML* anterior malleal ligament, *LML* lateral malleal ligament, *PIL* posterior incudal ligament, *TTM* tensor tympani muscle tendon, *CP* cochleariform process, *PE* pyramidal eminence, *LSCC* lateral semicircular canal, *PB* petrous bone

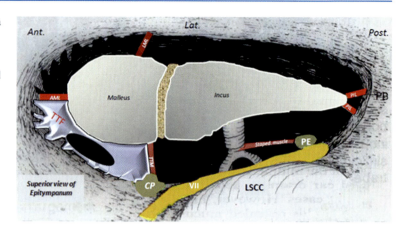

Fig. 3.40 Superior view of a right middle ear showing the tympanic diaphragm. *AMLF* anterior malleal ligamental fold, *TTF* tensor tympani fold, *LMF* lateral malleal fold, *LIMF* lateral incudomalleal fold, *AML* anterior malleal ligament, *LML* lateral malleal ligament, *PIL* posterior incudal ligament, *TTM* tensor tympani muscle tendon, *CP* cochleariform process, *PE* pyramidal eminence, *LSCC* lateral semicircular canal, *PB* petrous bone

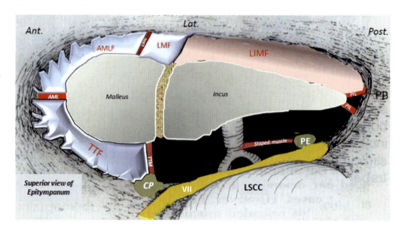

3.6.4   The Tympanic Isthmus

The mesotympanum connects with the Eustachian tube. However, the attic and the mastoid are isolated from the mesotympanum by the tympanic diaphragm. Attic aeration occurs through a 2.5-mm opening in the tympanic diaphragm called the tympanic isthmus (Fig. 3.41).

The entire attic is ventilated through the tympanic isthmus.

The Prussak's space is ventilated through the posterior pouch of von Tröltsch [65, 67].

The tympanic isthmus extends from the tensor tympani muscle anteriorly to the posterior incudal ligament posterosuperiorly and the pyramidal eminence posteroinferiorly. The distance from the TTM to the anterior edge of the posterior incudal ligament is around 6 mm [61]. The tympanic isthmus is limited medially by the attic bone and laterally by the body and short process of the incus and the head of the malleus.

The tympanic isthmus is divided by the medial incudal fold into two portions (Fig. 3.41).

3.6.4.1 The Anterior Tympanic Isthmus
The anterior tympanic isthmus, most important, is situated between the TTM anteriorly and the stapes posteroinferiorly. The diameter of this pathway is from 1 to 3 mm. It is a large open communication with the anterior epitympanum.

3.6.4.2 The Posterior Tympanic Isthmus
The posterior tympanic isthmus, less important, is situated between the short process of the incus and the stapedial muscle [65, 68].

Clinical Correlation
In long-standing chronic otitis media, granulation tissue and webs may block the tympanic isthmus and lead to failure of attic

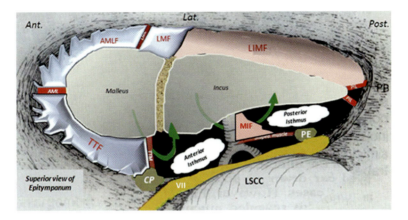

Fig. 3.41 Superior view of a right middle ear showing the tympanic diaphragm and the tympanic isthmus. The tympanic isthmus could be divided into anterior and posterior isthmus by the medial incudal fold (*MIF*). The *green arrows* represent the normal route of attic aeration from the mesotympanum. *AMLF* anterior malleal ligamental fold, *TTF* tensor tympani fold, *LMF* lateral malleal fold, *LIMF* lateral incudomalleal fold, *AML* anterior malleal ligament, *LML* lateral malleal ligament, *PIL* posterior incudal ligament, *TTM* tensor tympani muscle tendon, *CP* cochleariform process, *PE* pyramidal eminence, *LSCC* lateral semicircular canal, *PB* petrous bone

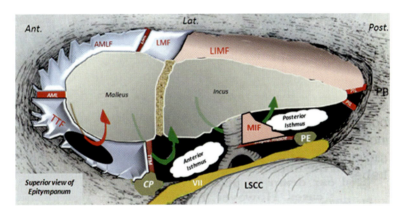

Fig. 3.42 Superior view of a right middle ear tympanic diaphragm showing a common variation of this structure. The tensor tympani fold (*TTF*) is incomplete and represents an accessory route of attic aeration (*red arrow*) from the protympanum. The *green arrows* represent the constant attic aeration through the tympanic isthmus. *AMLF* anterior malleal ligamental fold, *MIF* medial incudal fold, *LMF* lateral malleal fold, *LIMF* lateral incudomalleal fold, *AML* anterior malleal ligament, *LML* lateral malleal ligament, *PIL* posterior incudal ligament, *TTM* tensor tympani muscle tendon, *CP* cochleariform process, *PE* pyramidal eminence, *LSCC* lateral semicircular canal, *PB* petrous bone

ventilation even in the presence of a normally functioning Eustachian tube and well-aerated mesotympanum. This condition is called selective attic dysventilation and may result in chronic attical inflammation, attical retraction pockets, and attical cholesteatoma in the presence of a normal mesotympanum, and even in the presence of a tympanostomy tube (see Sect. 4.5.1.2 Clinical Applications).

Only a permanent large communication between the attic and the supratubal recess of the protympanum will guarantee the necessary aeration of the attic compartments to prevent attic dysventilation [69–71].

Incomplete TTF allows good ventilation from the protympanic space to the anterior attic and prevents attic dysventilation even in case of tympanic isthmus blockage. This confirms the importance of TTF removal during surgical treatment of middle ear disease to insure a good ventilation of the attic region [72–74] (Fig. 3.42).

References

1. Moore KL, Persaud TVN. The developing human: clinically oriented embryology. 5th ed. Philadelphia: W. B. Saunders Company; 1993.
2. le Douarin N, Kalcheim C. The neural crest. Cambridge: Cambridge University Press; 1999.
3. Keith A. Human embryology and morphology. London: Edward Arnold; 1948.
4. Baxter JS. Frazer's manual of embryology. 3rd ed. London: Baillière, Tindall & Cox; 1953. p. 202–5, 235–243.
5. Bast TH, Anson BJ, Richany SF. The development of the second branchial arch (Reichert's cartilage), facial canal and associated structures in man. Q Bull Northwest Univ Med Sch. 1956;30:235–49.
6. Anson BJ, Hanson JR, Richany SF. Early embryology of the auditory ossicles and associated structures in relation to certain anomalies observed clinically. Ann Otol. 1960;69:427–47.
7. Bastian D, Tran Ba Huy P. Organogenèse de l'oreille moyenne. Encycl Med Chir Paris: ORL. 1996; 20-005-A-30:4–12.
8. Nager GT. Aural atresia: anatomy and surgery. Postgrad Med. 1961;29:529–41.
9. Hough JV. Congenital malformations of the middle ear. Arch Otolaryngol. 1963;78:127–35.
10. Nomura Y, Nagao Y, Fukaya T. Anomalies of the middle ear. Laryngoscope. 1988;98:390–3.
11. Rahbar R, Neault MW, Kenna MA. Congenital absence of the incus bilaterally without other otologic anomalies: a new case report. Ear Nose Throat J. 2002;81:274–8.
12. Hanson JR, Anson BJ, Strickland EM. Branchial sources of the auditory ossicles in man: part II observation of embryonic stages from 7 mm to 28 mm (CR length). Arch Otolaryngol. 1962;76:200–15.
13. Louryan S. Développement des osselets de l'ouïe chez l'embryon humain: corrélation avec les données recueillies chez la souris. Bull Assoc Anat. 1993;77:29–32.
14. Louryan S, Glineur R. The mouse stapes develops mainly from the Reichert's cartilage independently of the otic capsule. Eur Arch Biol. 1993;103: 211–2.
15. Louryan S, Heymans O, J-C GOFFARD. Ear malformations in the mouse embryo after maternal administration of triazène, with clinical implications. Surg Radiol Anat. 1995;17:59–64.
16. Louryan S, Vanmuylder N, Resimont S. Ectopic stapes: a case report with embryologic correlations. Surg Radiol Anat. 2003;25:342–4.
17. Louryan S. Morphogénèse des osselets de l'oreille moyenne chez l'embryon des souris: I. Aspects morphologiques. Arch Biol. 1986;97:317–37.
18. Louryan S. In vitro development of mouse middle ear ossicles: a preliminary report. Eur Arch Biol. 1991; 102:55–8.
19. Jaskoll F. Morphogensis and teratogenesis of the middle ear in animals. Birth Defects Orig Artic Ser. 1980;XVI(7):9–28.
20. Jaskoll TF, Maderson PFA. A histological study of the development of the avian middle ear and tympanum. Anat Rec. 1978;190:177–99. doi:10.1002/ar.1091900203.
21. Anson BJ, Caulowell EW. The developmental anatomy of the human stapes. Ann Otol Rhinol Laryngol. 1942;51:891–904.
22. Rodriguez K, Shah RK, Kenna M. Anomalies of the middle and inner ear. Otolaryngol Clin North Am. 2007;40(1):81–96, vi. Review. PubMed PMID: 17346562.
23. Louryan S. Pure second branchial arch syndrome. Ann Otol Rhinol Laryngol. 1993;102:904–5.
24. Davies DG. Malleus fixation. J Laryngol Otol. 1968;82:331–51.
25. Martin JF, Bradley A, Olson EN. The paired-like homeo box gene MHox is required for early events of skeletogenesis in multiple lineages. Genes Dev. 1995;9:1237–49.
26. Funasaka S. Congenital ossicular anomalies without malformations of the external ear. Arch Otorhinolaryngol. 1979;224:231–40.
27. Tabb HG. Symposium: congenital anomalies of the middle ear. I. Epitympanic fixation of incus and malleus. Laryngoscope. 1976;86(2):243–6.
28. Mansour S, Nicolas K, Sbeity S. Triple ossicular fixation and semicircular canal malformations. J Otolaryngol. 2007;36(3):E31–4.
29. Kurosaki Y, Tanaka YO, Itai Y. Malleus bar as a rare cause of congenital malleus fixation: CT demonstration. AJNR Am J Neuroradiol. 1998;19:1229–30.
30. Carfrae MJ, Jahrsdoerfer RA, Kesser BW. Malleus bar: an unusual ossicular abnormality in the setting of congenital aural atresia. Otol Neurotol. 2010;31(3):415–8.
31. Nandapalan V, Tos M. Isolated congenital stapes ankylosis: an embryologic survey and literature review. Am J Otol. 2000;21(1):71–80.
32. Herman HK, Kimmelman CP. Congenital anomalies limited to the middle ear. Otolaryngol Head Neck Surg. 1992;106:285–7.
33. Swartz JD, Wolfson RJ, Marlowe FI, Popky GL. Postinflammatory ossicular fixation: CT analysis with surgical correlation. Radiology. 1985;154:697–700.
34. Chien W, Northrop C, Levine S, Pilch BZ, Peake WT, Rosowski JJ, et al. Anatomy of the distal incus in humans. J Assoc Res Otolaryngol. 2009;10(4):485–96.
35. Funnell W, Robert J, Heng Siah T, McKee Marc D, et al. On the coupling between the incus and the stapes in the cat. J Assoc Res Otolaryngol. 2005;6:9–18.
36. Watson C. Necrosis of the incus by the chorda tympani nerve. J Laryngol Otol. 1992;106:252–3.
37. Lannigan FJ, O'Higgins P, McPhie P. The vascular supply of the lenticular and long processes of the incus. Clin Otolaryngol Allied Sci. 1993;18:387–9.
38. Alberti PW. The blood supply of the long process of the incus and the head and neck of stapes. J Laryngol Otol. 1965;79:966–70.
39. aWengen DF, Nishihara S, Kurokawa H, Goode RL. Measurements of stapes superstructure. Ann Otol Rhinol Laryngol. 1995;104:311–6.

40. House JW. Otosclerosis. In: Hughes GB, Pensak ML, editors. Clinical otology. 2nd ed. New York: Thieme; 1997. p. 241–9.

41. Bruner H. Attachment of the stapes to the oval window in man. Arch Otolaryngol. 1954;50:18–29.

42. Whyte Orozco JR, Cisneros Gimeno AI, Yus Gotor C, Obón Nogues JA, Pérez Sanz R, Gañet Solé JF, et al. Ontogenic development of the incudostapedial joint. Acta Otorrinolaringol Esp. 2008;59(8):384–9.

43. Noden DM. The embryonic origins of the avian cephalic and cervical muscles and associated connective tissues. Am J Anat. 1983;168:257–76.

44. Kurosaki Y, Kuramoto K, Matsumoto K, Itai Y, Hara A, Kusukari J. Congenital ossification of the stapedius tendon: diagnosis with CT. Radiology. 1995;195:711–4.

45. Hough JV. Congenital malformation of the middle ear. Arch Otolaryngol. 1963;78:335–43.

46. Williams PL, Bannister LH, Berry MM, Collins P, Dyson M, Dussek JE, et al., editors. Gray's anatomy. 38th ed. New York: Churchill Livingstone Publishers; 1995. p. 263–84.

47. Wynsberghe DV, Noback CR, Carola R. The senses. In: Wynsberghe DV, Noback CR, Carola R, editors. Human anatomy and physiology. 3rd ed. New York: McGraw-Hill Inc; 1995. p. 512.

48. Glasscock ME, Gulya AJ. Developmental anatomy of the temporal bone and skull base. In: Gulya AJ, editor. Glasscock-Shambaugh surgery of the ear. 5th ed. Hamilton: BC Decker Inc; 2003. p. 19–25.

49. Moreano EH, Paparella MM, Zeltman D, Goycoolea MV. Prevalence of facial canal dehiscence and of persistent stapedial artery in the human middle ear: a report of 1000 temporal bones. Laryngoscope. 1994;104:309–20.

50. Steffen TN. Vascular anomalies of the middle ear. Laryngoscope. 1968;78:171–97.

51. David GD. Persistent stapedial artery: a temporal bone report. J Laryngol Otol. 1967;81:649–60.

52. Silbergleit R, Quint DJ, Mehta BA, et al. The persistent stapedial artery. Am J Neuroradiol. 2000;21:572. (Case series and review of persistent stapedial artery, with a detailed discussion of embryology and developmental anatomy). [PMID: 10730654].

53. Lasjaunias P, Moret J, Maelfe C. Arterial anomalies of the base of the skull. Neuroradiology. 1997;13:267–72.

54. Moret J. La vascularisation de l'appareil auditif. J Neuroradiol. 1982;9:209–60.

55. Hammar JA. Studien ueber die Entwicklung des Vorderdarms und einiger angrenzender Organe. Arch Mikrskop Anat. 1902;59:471–628.

56. Palva T, Ramsay H, Böhling T. Prussak's space revisited. Am J Otol. 1996;17(4):512–20.

57. Palva T, Ramsay H. Aeration of Prussak's space is independent of the supradiaphragmatic epitympanic compartments. Otol Neurotol. 2007;28(2):264–8.

58. Von Tröltsch A. Lehrbuch der Ohrenheilkunde mit Einschluss der anatomie des Ohres. 7th ed. Leipzig: FCW Vogel; 1881.

59. Helmholtz H. Eine kiirzlich in der Zeitschrift ftir rationelle Medicin, in Archiv für die gesamte Physiologie des Menschen und der Tiere 1868. vol 1, Issue 1. Germany: Springer; 1868. p. 1–60.

60. Prussak A. Zur Anatomie des menschlichen Trommelfells. Arch Ohrenheilkd. 1867;3:255–78.

61. Palva T, Johnsson LG. Epitympanic compartment surgical considerations: reevaluation. Am J Otol. 1995;16(4):505–13.

62. Onal K, Haastert RM, Grote JJ. Structural variations of supratubal recess: the anterior epitympanic space. Am J Otol. 1997;18:317–21.

63. Palva T, Ramsay H, Bohlurg J. Lateral and anterior view to tensor fold and supratubal recess. Am J Otol. 1998;19:405–14.

64. Chatellier HP, Lemoine J. Le diaphragme interatticotympanique du nouveau-nÈ. Description de sa morphologie; considÈrations sur son rÙle pathogÈnique dans les oto-mastoÔdites cloisonnÈes du nourrisson. Ann Otolaryngol Chir Cervicofac (Paris). 1946; 13:534–66.

65. Palva T, Ramsay H. Incudal folds and epitympanic aeration. Am J Otol. 1996;17:700–8.

66. Palva T, Ramsay H, Böhling T. Tensor fold and anterior epitympanum. Am J Otol. 1997;18:307–16.

67. Chatelliere HP, Lemoine J. Le diaphragme interatticotympanique du nouveau-ne´. Ann Otolaryngol Chir Cervicofac. 1946;13:534–66.

68. Proctor B. The development of the middle ear spaces and their surgical significance. J Laryngol Otol. 1964;78:631–48.

69. Palva T, Ramsay H. Chronic inflammatory ear disease and cholesteatoma: creation of auxiliary attic aeration pathways by microdissection. Am J Otol. 1999;20(2): 145–51.

70. Marchioni D, Alicandri-Ciufelli M, Molteni G, Artioli FL, Genovese E, Presutti L. Selective epitympanic dysventilation syndrome. Laryngoscope. 2010;120(5): 1028–33.

71. Marchioni D, Grammatica A, Alicandri-Ciufelli M, Aggazzotti-Cavazza E, Genovese E, Presutti L. The contribution of selective dysventilation to attical middle ear pathology. Med Hypotheses. 2011;77(1): 116–20.

72. Palva T, Böhling T, Ramsay H. Attic aeration in temporal bones from children with recurring otitis media: tympanostomy tubes did not cure disease in Prussak's space. Am J Otol. 2000;21:485–93.

73. Mansour S, Nicolas K, Naim A, et al. Inflammatory chronic otitis media and the anterior epitympanic recess. J Otolaryngol. 2005;34:149–58.

74. Marchioni D, Alicandri-Ciufelli M, Grammatica A, Mattioli F, Genovese E, Presutti L. Lateral endoscopic approach to epitympanic diaphragm and Prussak's space: a dissection study. Surg Radiol Anat. 2010;32(9): 843–52.

75. Tos M. Manual of middle ear surgery and reconstructive procedures, vol. 2. New York: Thieme publishers; 1995.

76. Marchioni D. Lateral endoscopic approach to epitympanic diaphragm and Prussak's space: a dissection study. Surg Radiol Anat. 2010;32(9):843–52.

Middle Ear Compartments

4

Contents

The middle ear cavity is anatomically not only a sole chamber, but a space with different compartments. The objective of this chapter is to present a detailed and exhaustive description of these compartments, their frontiers, their relationship, and their connections to improve the understanding of the pathophysiology of the inflammatory and cholesteatomatous middle ear diseases.

The middle ear cavity was divided into five compartments: the mesotympanum in the center, the epitympanum superiorly, the protympanum anteriorly, the hypotympanum inferiorly, and the retrotympanum posteriorly (Fig. 4.1).

In addition, this chapter, based on the description of the anatomy of the middle ear folds in Chap. 3, will describe several anatomo-functional units inside or even beyond the traditional division of the compartments.

The comprehensive knowledge of this detailed anatomy is the key of success in the management of middle ear disorders.

4.1 Embryology of Middle Ear Compartments

In the developing human, the tympanomastoid system appears in the 3rd week of life from an outpouching of the first pharyngeal pouch called the tubotympanic recess. The endodermal tissue of the dorsal end of this pouch becomes the Eustachian tube and the tympanic cavity [1].

By the 7th week, a concomitant growth of the second branchial arch constricts the midportion of

S. Mansour et al., *Comprehensive and Clinical Anatomy of the Middle Ear*,
DOI 10.1007/978-3-642-36967-4_4, © Springer-Verlag Berlin Heidelberg 2013

the tubotympanic recess, placing the primary tympanic cavity lateral to this constriction and the primordial Eustachian tube medial to this constriction [1]. The future development of the Eustachian tube is marked by lengthening, narrowing, and mesodermal chondrification establishing the fibrocartilaginous Eustachian tube (see Sect. 7.1).

The terminal end of the tubotympanic recess buds into four sacci: the saccus anticus, the sac-

cus medius, the saccus superior, and the saccus posticus [1–3]. These sacci expand progressively to replace middle ear mesenchyme and mastoid mesenchyme (Fig. 4.2). The walls of the expanding sacci envelop the ossicular chain and line the walls of middle ear cavity; the interface between two sacci gives rise to several mesentery-like mucosal folds, transmitting blood vessels and ligaments to middle ear contents.

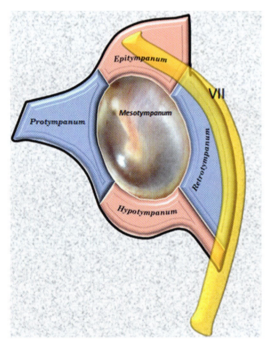

Fig. 4.1 Middle ear compartments; *VII* facial nerve

4.1.1 The Saccus Anticus

The saccus anticus is the smallest saccus. It extends upward anterior to the tensor tympani tendon to form the anterior epitympanic recess and the anterior pouch of von Tröltsch. At the level of the tensor tympani muscle canal, it fuses with the anterior saccule of the saccus medius to form an important mucosal fold, the tensor tympani fold. The tensor tympani fold separates the anterior epitympanic recess superiorly from the supratubal recess inferiorly [2] (Figs. 4.2 and 4.3).

4.1.2 The Saccus Medius

The saccus medius forms the attic. It extends upward and divides into three saccules:
1. Anterior saccule: It develops upward to form the anterior compartment of the attic.
2. Medial saccule: The medial saccule forms the superior incudal space by its growth over

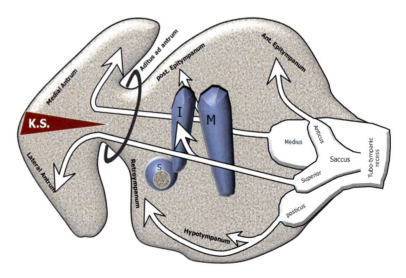

Fig. 4.2 Embryology of middle ear spaces. *I* incus, *M* malleus; S, stapes, *KS* Korner's septum

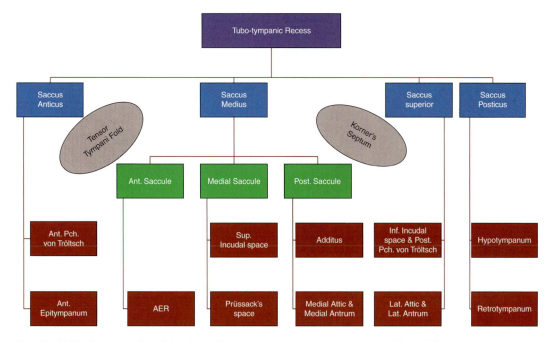

Fig. 4.3 Table illustrating the origin of the different spaces, recesses, and pouches of the middle ear

the incudomalleal bodies and the posterior incudal ligament. The medial saccule sends an offshoot forward to form the Prussak's space.

3. Posterior saccule: The posterior saccule extends posteriorly between the long process of the incus and the stapes to form the medial portion of the mastoid antrum which is derived from the petrous part of the temporal bone [2] (Figs. 4.2 and 4.3).

4.1.3   The Saccus Superior

The saccus superior forms the posterior pouch of von Tröltsch and the inferior incudal space. It extends posteriorly and laterally between the handle of the malleus and the long process of the incus to form the posterior pouch of von Tröltsch, the inferior incudal space, and the lateral part of the antrum which derives from the squamous part of the temporal bone.

The plane of fusion between the posterior saccule of the saccus medius, which forms the medial part of mastoid air cells system, and the saccus superior, which forms the lateral part of mastoid air cells system, usually breaks down. If the breakdown fails, a bony septum persists between

the two parts, called the Korner's septum [2] (Figs. 4.2 and 4.3).

4.1.4   The Saccus Posticus

The saccus posticus extends along the hypotympanum and rises up posteriorly to form the round window niche, the oval window niche, the facial recess, and the sinus tympani.

The sinus tympani has a variable size and depth posteriorly; this variation is dependent on the degree of extension of the saccus posticus under the stapedial tendon during fetal development [2] (Figs. 4.2 and 4.3).

4.2   Anatomy of the Protympanum

The protympanum is the middle ear compartment that lies anterior to a frontal plane drawn through the anterior margin of the tympanic annulus (Fig. 4.1). This space is widely open posteriorly into the mesotympanum; it leads anteriorly into the Eustachian tube. We included into the protympanum the whole bony portion of the Eustachian tube which is 1 cm long in adults.

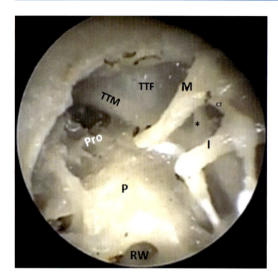

Fig. 4.4 Endoscopic view of a left cadaveric middle ear showing the protympanum (*Pro*) which is limited superiorly by the canal of the tensor tympani muscle (*TTM*) and the tensor tympani fold (*TTF*). (*) cochleariform process, *M* malleus, *I* incus, *P* promontory, *RW* round window, *CT* chorda tympani

4.2.1   Walls of the Protympanum

The lateral wall of the protympanum consists of a thin plate of the tympanic bone called the lateral lamina; this plate separates the protympanum from the mandibular fossa. The medial wall consists of the cochlea posteriorly and the carotid canal anteriorly. The roof is composed of the bony semicanal for the tensor tympani muscle and the tensor tympani fold separating the protympanum from the anterior attic (Fig. 4.4).

4.2.2   The Supratubal Recess (STR)

The supratubal recess is the superior extension of the protympanum. It corresponds to the space lying between the superior border of the tympanic orifice of the Eustachian tube and the tensor tympani fold. It lies below the anterior attic from which it is separated by the tensor tympani fold (TTF).

The size of the supratubal recess depends on the anatomy of the TTF (see Sect. 3.6.2.10). The

TTF forms the roof of the protympanum and has variable orientations depending on the level of its anterior insertion. For instance, a horizontal TTF results in a small or even absent supratubal recess and a vertical TTF gives place to a large supratubal recess [4–6] (see Fig. 3.38).

4.3   Anatomy of the Hypotympanum

The hypotympanum is a crescent-shaped space located at the bottom of the middle ear. It lies below a horizontal plane starting from the inferior margin of the fibrous annulus to the inferior margin of cochlear promontory; it is surrounded by five walls.

4.3.1   Walls of the Hypotympanum

- *The anterior wall* is formed by the carotid canal medially and by a dense bone laterally.
- *The posterior wall* is formed by the inferior part of the styloid complex and the vertical segment of the facial nerve canal. Frequently, the posterior wall is pneumatized by air cells (retrofacial air cells) which extend from the mastoid antrum to the hypotympanum medial to the facial nerve. The posterior wall corresponds to a vertical plane from the posterior semicircular canal to the junction of the sigmoid sinus with the jugular bulb.
- *The outer wall* is formed by the tympanic bone.
- *The medial wall* is formed by the lower part of the promontory and a part of the petrous bone which extends under the promontory. This wall is usually pneumatized; its air cell system may extend beneath the cochlea to reach the petrous apex air cells. Rarely the medial wall is compact (Fig. 4.5).
- *The inferior wall* corresponds to a thin bony plate separating the hypotympanum from the jugular bulb (Fig. 4.5). In cases of a high jugular bulb, the hypotympanum is significantly reduced, or it could even be missing.

Fig. 4.5 Endoscopic view of a left ear showing the hypotympanum and some hypotympanic cells. Notice that the hypotympanum lies below the level of the tympanic sulcus (*S*). In this case, the inferior wall of the hypotympanum is smooth and consists of a thin plate of bone separating the middle ear from the jugular bulb. *RW* round window

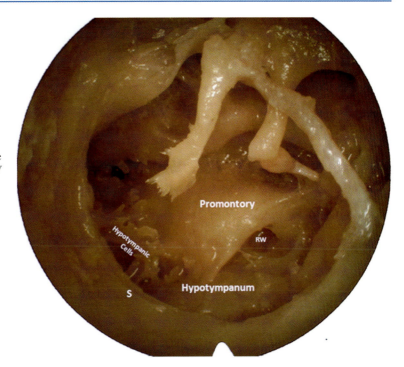

4.3.2   Air Cells in the Hypotympanum

The air cells of the hypotympanum are divided into:

4.3.2.1 Hypotympanic Air Cells

The hypotympanic air cells, present in the medial and inferior wall of the hypotympanum, may extend below the labyrinth to reach the petrous apex cells (infralabyrinthine tract) (Fig. 4.6 and see Fig. 2.12b).

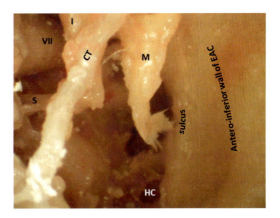

Fig. 4.6 Endoscopic view of a right ear showing hypotympanic cells in the inferior and medial wall of the hypotympanum. *M* malleus, *I* incus, *S* stapes, *CT* chorda tympani, *VII* tympanic segment of the facial nerve

Surgical Applications

Infracochlear Approach

Through a transcanal hypotympanotomy, removal of the bone and the cells of the medial wall of the hypotympanum, between the carotid artery anteriorly and the jugular bulb posteriorly, offers a direct surgical approach for the drainage of the petrous apex [7–9].

4.3.2.2 Retrofacial Cells

The retrofacial cells extend from the central mastoid tract medial to the facial nerve and drain into the hypotympanic space.

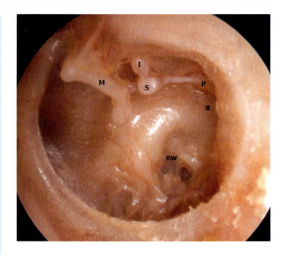

Fig. 4.7 Otoscopic view of a left ear showing adhesive otitis media and a posterior pars tensa retraction pocket into the retrotympanum (*). *I* incus with lysis of its long process, *M* malleus, *S* stapes, *P* pyramidal eminence, *RW* round window

4.4 Anatomy of the Retrotympanum

The retrotympanum is a complex region. It consists of several separate spaces lying in the posterior aspect of the tympanic cavity medial and posterior to the tympanic annulus (Fig. 4.1). The retrotympanum is the site of the highest incidence of middle ear pathologies especially retraction pockets and cholesteatoma (Fig. 4.7).

The retrotympanum includes four spaces: two spaces lie medial to the vertical segment of the facial nerve and the pyramidal eminence and two spaces lie lateral to them. These spaces are separated from each other by the bridges and the eminences of the posterior wall of the middle ear cavity. The pyramidal eminence is the fulcrum of the retrotympanum (Fig. 4.8) (see Sect. 2.3.2).

4.4.1 The Lateral Spaces

The lateral spaces of the retrotympanum form the facial recess. The facial recess is bordered medially by the facial canal and the pyramidal eminence and laterally by the chorda tympani. Superiorly, the facial recess is bounded by the incudal buttress, bony boundary of the incudal fossa, which lodges the short process of the incus. The incudal buttress separates the facial recess from the aditus ad antrum. Inferiorly, the facial recess is limited

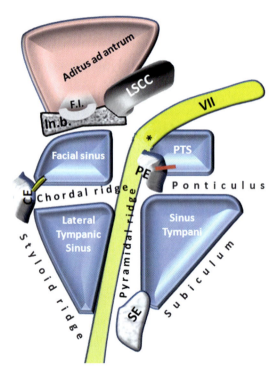

Fig. 4.8 Schematic drawing of the retrotympanum as viewed from the mesotympanum. *PE* pyramidal eminence, *CE* chordal eminence, *SE* styloid eminence, *VII* tympanic segment of facial nerve, * second genu of facial nerve, *FI* fossa incudis. *In.b.* incudal buttress, *PTS* posterior tympanic sinus, *LSCC* lateral semicircular canal

by the chordo-facial angle which ranges from 18° to 30°; the distance between the origin of the chorda tympani and the short process of the incus ranges from 5 to 10 mm [11].

The facial recess size is variable among individuals; however, it does not differ between age groups ranging from newborns to adults, indicating that it is near adult size at birth [12–14]. It measures about 2 mm at the level of the round window and 3 mm at the level of the oval window [15, 16].

The chordal ridge, which runs between the pyramidal eminence and the chordal eminence, divides the facial recess into the facial sinus superiorly and the lateral tympanic sinus inferiorly.

4.4.1.1 The Facial Sinus

The facial sinus is the superior part of the facial recess. It is a small pouch that is situated between the incudal buttress superiorly, the chordal ridge inferiorly, and the second genu of the facial nerve medially. There is no connection of the facial sinus with the air cells of the attic or mastoid process.

4.4.1.2 The Lateral Tympanic Sinus

The lateral tympanic sinus is the inferior part of the facial recess and is the most lateral and narrowest sinus of the retrotympanum. It represents the interval among the three eminences of the styloid complex (pyramidal eminence, styloid eminence, chordal eminence). It lies medial to the chordal eminence, inferior and lateral to the pyramidal eminence, and superior to the styloid eminence. The dimensions of the lateral tympanic sinus vary from 1.5 to 2.5 mm [17, 18]; it has no connection with the attic or the antrum.

Surgical Application

The facial recess serves as a posterior window to reach the middle ear from the mastoid cavity, enabling the visualization of the oval window and ponticulus superiorly and the round window and subiculum inferiorly. This important surgical approach is called transmastoid posterior tympanotomy; it is done by a transmastoid drilling of the posterior wall of the facial recess, between the chorda tympani laterally and the facial nerve medially (Fig. 4.9).

In cases of narrow facial recess or incomplete exposure of the target middle ear structure, extended facial recess approach could be done. In this technique, the chorda tympani nerve is sacrificed and drilling is done between the annulus of the

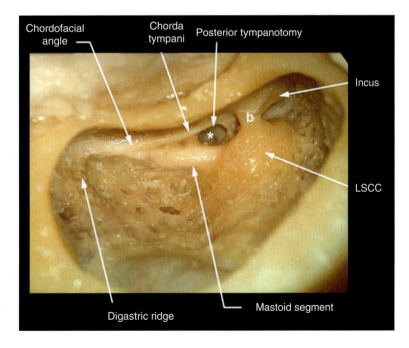

Fig. 4.9 Left ear, transmastoid posterior tympanotomy (*). *b* incudal buttress, *LSSC* lateral semicircular canal

Chordofacial angle

Chorda tympani

Posterior tympanotomy

Incus

LSCC

Digastric ridge

Mastoid segment

tympanic membrane and the facial nerve. This leads to a wider exposure of the middle ear. The mean width of the extended facial recess is about 5 mm [19, 20].

During posterior tympanotomy, the risk of facial nerve damage and the probability of sacrificing the chorda tympani depend on the dimensions of the facial recess [11, 18, 21, 22], which varies widely in the general population. However, preoperative thin-section CT scans allow surgeons to make a precise assessment of these anatomic structures during preoperative planning (Fig. 4.10).

4.4.2 The Medial Spaces

The medial spaces of the retrotympanum, called the tympanic sinus, are the depressions in the posterior wall of the middle ear that lie between the facial nerve and pyramidal eminence laterally and the labyrinth medially (Figs. 4.8 and 4.11).

The ponticulus, which runs from the promontory to the pyramidal eminence, divides the tympanic sinus in two spaces: the posterior

tympanic sinus superiorly and the sinus tympani inferiorly.

4.4.2.1 Posterior Tympanic Sinus

The posterior tympanic sinus is present in most middle ears [23]; it lies superior to the ponticulus, medial to the pyramidal eminence and facial nerve. It is about 1 mm deep and about 1.5 mm long [24]. In ears where the ponticulus does not reach the posterior wall of the middle ear, the posterior tympanic sinus merges with the sinus tympani to form one confluent sinus.

> **Surgical Application**
> During middle ear surgery, in order to reach the posterior tympanic sinus, section of the stapedial tendon and drilling of the pyramidal process may be required.

4.4.2.2 The Sinus Tympani

The sinus tympani is the largest sinus of the retrotympanum. It lies medial to the mastoid portion of the facial nerve, lateral to the posterior semicircular canal. It is limited superiorly by the

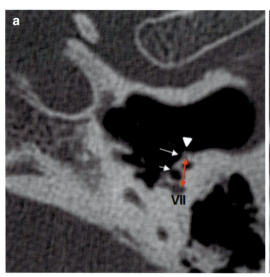
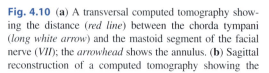
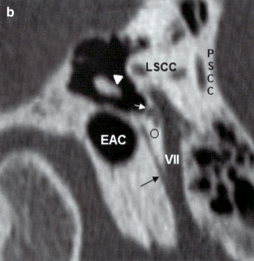

Fig. 4.10 (**a**) A transversal computed tomography showing the distance (*red line*) between the chorda tympani (*long white arrow*) and the mastoid segment of the facial nerve (*VII*); the *arrowhead* shows the annulus. (**b**) Sagittal reconstruction of a computed tomography showing the emergence of the chorda (*black arrow*) from the facial nerve (*VII*) and the bony wall (*circle*) between the chorda and the VII (facial recess approach). *White arrow* facial recess, *white arrowhead* short process of the incus, *LSCC* lateral semicircular canal, *PSCC* posterior semicircular canal

ponticulus and the pyramidal eminence and inferiorly by the subiculum and the styloid eminence.

The sinus tympani has a great variability in size and shape and depth. Its posterior extension varies between 0.2 and 10 mm with an average of 2 mm [25–27].

In about 10 % of the population, the sinus tympani and posterior tympanic sinus form one confluent recess [24].

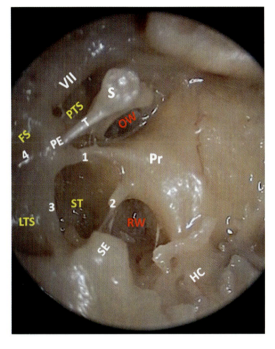

Fig. 4.11 Endoscopic view of a right middle ear showing the different sinuses and recesses of the retrotympanum. *PTS* posterior tympanic sinus, *ST* sinus tympani, *LTS* lateral tympanic sinus, *FS* facial sinus, *PE* pyramidal eminence, *SE* styloid eminence, *1* ponticulus, *2* subiculum, *3* pyramidal ridge, *4* chordal ridge, *OW* oval window, *RW* round window, *S* stapes, *T* stapedial tendon, *Pr* promontory, *HC* hypotympanic cells, *VII* facial nerve

Sinus Tympani Types and Surgical Approaches

Based on its depth, the sinus tympani is classified into three types with an equal frequency in the general population [28, 29] (Fig. 4.12).

- Type A is a shallow sinus tympani; it is small and does not reach the level of the vertical portion of the facial nerve posteriorly. In such cases surgical transcanal access to the sinus tympani is possible.
- Type B sinus tympani is of intermediate depth; it lies medial to the vertical portion of the facial nerve but does not extend posteriorly deeper than the level of the facial nerve. A total and clear visualization of such sinus tympani could not be achieved without the use of an endoscope. Any blind dissection in the sinus tympani without endoscopic visualization carries a risk of residual disease or a possible injury to a dehiscent facial nerve or a high jugular bulb [30].

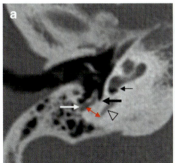 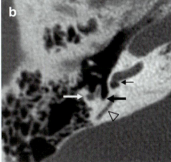 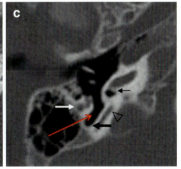

Fig. 4.12 Transversal computed tomographic view of right ears with different depths of the sinus tympani. (**a**) Type A, (**b**) Type B, (**c**) Type C. Deepest point of the sinus tympani (*thick black arrow*), facial nerve (*white arrow*), round window membrane (*thin black arrow*), posterior semicircular canal PSCC (*arrowhead*). The *red arrow* in (**a**) represents the distance between the facial nerve and the PSCC. The *red arrow* in (**c**) represents the retrofacial approach to the sinus tympani

- Type C sinus tympani is very deep; it extends posteriorly more deeply than the vertical portion of the facial nerve. This type is frequently encountered in a well-pneumatized mastoid. Despite the use of an otoendoscope, the pathology of such deep sinus could not be explored entirely from the middle ear; therefore, access should be obtained through a transmastoid retrofacial approach. This approach requires enough distance of more than 2 mm between the facial nerve and the posterior semicircular canal; otherwise, these structures could be easily injured.

4.5   Anatomy of the Attic (The Epitympanum)

The attic is the part of the tympanum situated above an imaginary plane passing through the short process of the malleus. The attic occupies approximately one-third of the vertical dimension of the entire tympanic cavity and lodges the head and neck of the malleus, the body, and the short process of the incus (Fig. 4.13). The attic is bounded by the following walls:

- *The lateral wall* of the attic is formed inferiorly by Shrapnell's membrane and superiorly by a bony wall, called the outer attic wall, "*le mur de la logette des osselets.*"
- *The medial wall* of the attic is a part of the medial wall situated above the tympanic segment of the facial nerve and tensor tympani muscle. It contains the lateral semicircular canal. This wall may be pneumatized by the supralabyrinthine tract (see Sect. 2.6.2 and Fig. 2.33).
- *The posterior wall* is occupied almost entirely by the aditus ad antrum. It is 5–6 mm high and is usually larger above than below. The aditus provides a communication between the antrum and the rest of the tympanic cavity.
- *Inferiorly*, the tympanic diaphragm divides the attic into an upper unit situated above the

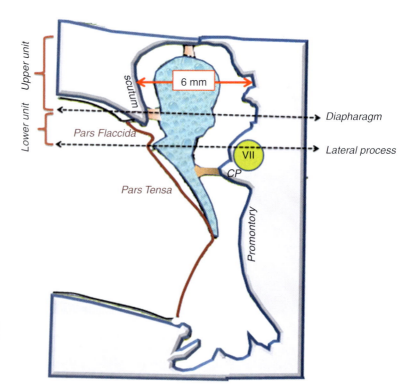

Fig. 4.13 Schema showing the upper unit and the lower unit of the attic. *VII* facial nerve, *CP* cochleariform process

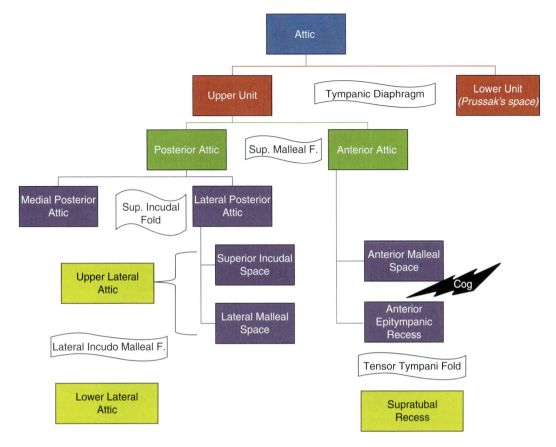

Fig. 4.14 Table showing the organization of the different compartments of the attic

tympanic diaphragm and a lower unit of the attic (the Prussak's space), which is below the diaphragm. Medially, the tympanic diaphragm separates the upper unit of the attic from the underlying upper mesotympanum. The upper unit of the attic and the mesotympanum communicate together for ventilation purposes through an opening through the diaphragm called the tympanic isthmus [33, 34] (Figs. 4.13 and 4.14) (see Sect. 3.6.3).

4.5.1   The Upper Unit of the Attic

The upper unit of the attic lies above the tympanic diaphragm (see Chap. 3, Mucosal Folds). Medially, the tympanic diaphragm separates the upper unit of the attic completely from the

underlying upper mesotympanum. A communication between both spaces for ventilation purposes is only possible through an opening of the tympanic diaphragm, called the *tympanic isthmus* (see Fig. 3.41). The tympanic isthmus is situated between the tensor tympani muscle anteriorly and the posterior incudal ligament posteriorly (see Sect. 3.6.4) Laterally, the tympanic diaphragm separates the upper unit of the attic from the lower unit of the attic, the Prussak's space. Posteriorly, the upper unit of the attic communicates with the mastoid cavity through the aditus ad antrum.

In addition to this separation by the tympanic diaphragm in the horizontal plane, several folds and ligaments in the perpendicular planes lead to further divisions and spaces of the upper unit of the attic:

Fig. 4.15 Superior view of a right middle ear, showing the attic divided by the superior malleal fold (*SMF*) into a smaller anterior attic and a larger posterior attic. *AML* anterior malleal ligament, *LML* lateral malleal ligament, *TTM* tensor tympani muscle tendon, *PB* petrous bone, *PIL* posterior incudal ligament, *PE* pyramidal eminence, *CP* cochleariform process, *VII* facial nerve, *LSCC* lateral semicircular canal

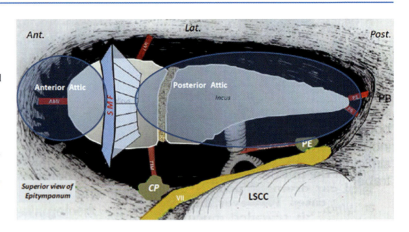

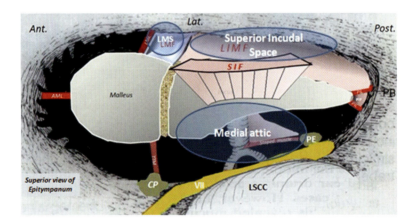

Fig. 4.16 Superior view of the right middle ear, showing the different compartments of the posterior attic. The medial attic lies medial to the superior incudal fold (*SIF*), the superior incudal space lies above the lateral incudomalleal fold (LIMF) and superior to SIF, the lateral malleal space (*LMS*) lies above the lateral malleal fold (*LMF*).

MIF medial incudal fold, *AML* anterior malleal ligament, *LML* lateral malleal ligament, *TTM* tensor tympani muscle, *PB* petrous bone, *PIL* posterior incudal ligament, *PE* pyramidal eminence, *CP* cochleariform process, *VII* facial nerve, *LSCC* lateral semicircular canal

The *superior malleal fold* with a coronal orientation divides the upper unit of the attic into two different spaces: a posterior and larger one, *the posterior attic*, and an anterior and smaller one, *the anterior attic* (Figs. 4.14 and 4.15).

4.5.1.1 Posterior Attic or Posterior Epitympanum

The posterior attic is largely occupied by the posterior part of the head of the malleus, the body, and short process of the incus. In adult, the distance from the tip of the incus to the attic roof is about 6 mm [31].

The posterior attic is divided into the medial posterior attic and the lateral posterior attic by the

superior incudal fold oriented in a sagittal plane (Figs. 4.14 and 4.16).

The Medial Posterior Attic

The medial posterior attic or the medial incudal space is the larger compartment of the posterior attic; it is bounded by the lateral semicircular canal and the Fallopian canal medially and the ossicles and the superior incudal fold laterally. The distance between the lateral semicircular canal and the incus body is 1.7 mm [33]. The medial posterior attic contains essentially the tympanic isthmus that is divided by the medial incudal fold into an anterior and a posterior tympanic isthmus. These openings represent the main

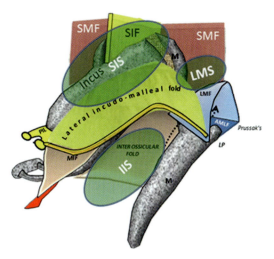

Fig. 4.17 Lateral view of a right middle ear after removal of the tympanic membrane and the outer attic wall, showing the different compartments of the lateral attic: the superior incudal space (*SIS*) above the lateral incudomalleal fold (*LIMF*), the inferior incudal space below the LIMF, and the lateral malleal space (*LMS*) above the lateral malleal fold (*LMF*) on a more inferior level than the SIS, but usually in open communication with each other. The posterior boundary of the LMS is represented by the descending portion of the LIMF. *SMF* superior malleal fold, *SIF* superior incudal fold, *PIL* posterior incudal ligament, *MIF* medial incudal fold, *M* malleus, *LP* lateral process of malleus, *AMLF* anterior malleal ligamental fold

route of aeration of the whole epitympanum (Figs. 4.14 and 4.16).

The Lateral Posterior Attic

The lateral posterior attic is narrower, located between the outer attic wall laterally and the malleus head, incus body, and superior incudal fold medially. The lateral posterior attic is further divided into three spaces: the superior incudal space and the lateral malleal space forming the upper lateral attic and the inferior incudal space, called the lower lateral attic (Figs. 4.14 and 4.16).

Upper Lateral Attic

The upper lateral attic is composed of two spaces that are largely opened to each other, but at different levels: posteriorly the space lying above the lateral incudomalleal fold is called the superior incudal space, and more anteriorly the

space lying above the lateral malleal fold is called the lateral malleal space (Figs. 4.14, 4.16, and 4.17).

- *Superior incudal space (SIS)*
The superior incudal space lies in a more superior position in relation to the lateral malleal space. It is limited inferiorly by the incudomalleolar fold which separates it from the inferior incudal space (Figs. 4.14, 4.16, and 4.17).

- *The lateral malleal space (LMS)*
The lateral malleal space is a distinct anatomic area, part of the lateral attic, and lies above the lateral malleal fold. It is limited medially by the malleus head and neck, laterally by the outer attic wall, anteriorly by the anterior malleal fold, and posteriorly by the downwards turning end of the incudomalleal fold [32]. The lateral malleal space is regularly opened superiorly and thus in free communication with the superior incudal space (Figs. 4.14, 4.16, and 4.17).

Infrequently, the lateral malleal fold is incomplete and a direct communication exists between the Prussak's space and the lateral malleal space [33–37].

In rare cases the incudomalleal fold may extend over the entire lateral malleal space; that means that the lateral incudomalleal fold slopes down and joins the posterior malleal fold. In such cases, the lateral malleal space is isolated, separated from the superior incudal space, but it gets in direct communication with the inferior incudal space [32].

Lower Lateral Attic: Inferior Incudal Space (IIS)

The inferior incudal space lies below the lateral incudomalleal fold, therefore inferior to the tympanic diaphragm. It is located between the more dependent portion of the short process and the body of the incus medially and the scutum laterally (Figs. 4.14 and 4.17). A particular region of the mesotympanum guarantees the ventilation of this space. This region of ventilation for the inferior incudal space is limited medially by the medial incudal fold and anteriorly by the interossicular fold which lies between the long process of the incus and the upper 2/3 of the malleus handle [31].

Fig. 4.18 Schema
of a medial view of a right
middle ear showing the
different spaces of the
anterior attic: *1* supratubal
recess, *TTF* tensor tympani
fold, *2* anterior epitympanic
recess, *3* anterior malleal
space, TTM tensor tympani
muscle (Reproduced with
permission from the Journal
of Otolaryngology-Head
And Neck Surgery, Decker
Publishing Publisher [43])

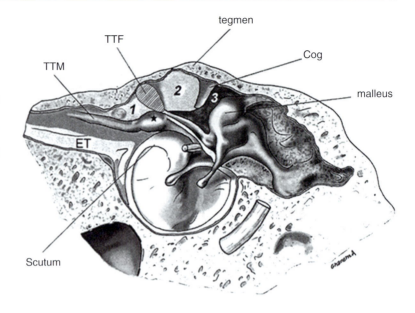

4.5.1.2 Anterior Attic or Anterior Epitympanum

The anterior attic is a separate cavity of varying shape. It is situated anterior to the head of malleus and the superior malleal fold.

The anterior epitympanum is divided into two spaces by the cog [36]. The cog is a bony crest that extends inferiorly from the tegmen; it is superior to the cochleariform process and anterosuperior to the malleus head. It divides the anterior attic into a small posterior space, the anterior malleal space, and large anterior space: the anterior epitympanic recess (Figs. 4.14, 4.15, and 4.18).

The Anterior Malleal Space (AMS)

The anterior malleal space is of variable size and situated between the head of the malleus posteriorly and the cog anteriorly (Figs. 4.14 and 4.18).

The Anterior Epitympanic Recess (AER)
(Figs. 4.14 and 4.18)

The anterior epitympanic recess has been given different names such as anterior epitympanic sinus, anterior epitympanic space, sinus epitym-

pani, and even supratubal recess. However, additional anatomic studies identified the supratubal recess (STR) and the anterior epitympanic recess (AER) as two distinct spaces separated by the tensor tympani fold (TTF) [6, 31, 37]. Therefore, the term anterior epitympanum should be reserved for the whole anatomic entity composed of the anterior malleal space and the AER. The supratubal recess is considered as a part of the protympanum (see Sect. 4.2.2).

The AER presents the following boundaries [37–39]:
- *Superiorly*: the anterior part of the tegmen tympani
- *Anteriorly*: the zygomatic root
- *Posteriorly*: the cog
- *Laterally*: the scutum
- *Medially*: the anterior portion of the tympanic portion of the facial nerve and the geniculate ganglion
- *The floor*: represented by the cochleariform process and the TTF (Fig. 4.18).

The TTF is an integral part of the tympanic diaphragm (see Sect. 3.6.3). When the TTF is complete, the anterior tympanic recess and the supratubal recess form two separate spaces. When there is a defect in the TTF (in 15 % of

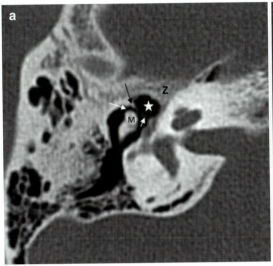
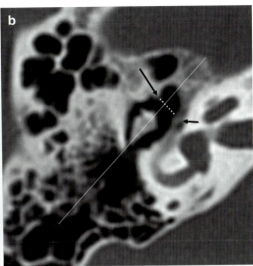

Fig. 4.19 Axial computed tomographic views of the anterior epitympanum. (**a**) The cog with its largest lateral part (*black arrow*) and its continuity towards the medial attic wall (*small white arrow*); anterior malleal space (*white long arrow*); anterior epitympanic recess AER (***); *M* malleus head, *Z* zygoma. (**b**) Mensuration of the relevant transversal diameter of the AER (*punctated line*), perpendicular to the incudo-malleal axis (*long white line*) between the lateral limit of the cog (*long black arrow*) and the cochleariform process (*short black arrow*)

cases), the AER is in direct communication with the supratubal recess serving as an accessory route of aeration of the attic called the anterior route of ventilation, the posterior route being represented by the anterior and posterior tympanic isthmus [35, 36, 38].

The size of the AER is variable between individuals. CT scan permits the measurement of the size of the recess; its mean size is about 4×4 mm. Transmastoid approach to the AER with conservation of the ossicular chain requires minimum dimensions of 3×3 mm [37] (Fig. 4.19).

recurs despite repetitive myringotomies with tube insertion. In addition the AER must be investigated in the presence of retraction pocket especially when it is anterosuperiorly oriented. In these cases the TTF is complete and blocks the aeration of the anterior epitympanum from the anterosuperior mesotympanum creating a dysventilation syndrome. This situation will not respond to posterior atticotomy alone.

When performing middle ear surgery for dysventilation pathology with isthmus blockage, an imaging study of the AER with CT scan is mandatory not only to assess its involvement but also to obtain its dimensions in order to select the surgical approach. Resection of the cog and the TTF is fundamental to create an anterior route of ventilation between the protympanum, the supratubal recess, the AER, and the posterior attic [35, 37].

Clinical Applications

The AER in Chronic Otitis Media (Fig. 4.20)
The AER is highly important to consider in cases of recurrent otorrhea with central or anterior perforation not responding to conventional medical therapy or in front of mucoid middle ear effusion that persists or

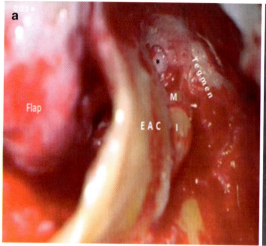
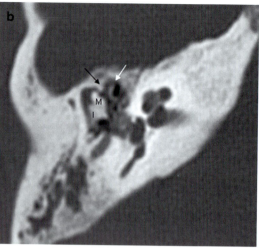
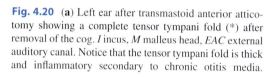

Fig. 4.20 (**a**) Left ear after transmastoid anterior attico-tomy showing a complete tensor tympani fold (*) after removal of the cog. *I* incus, *M* malleus head, *EAC* external auditory canal. Notice that the tensor tympani fold is thick and inflammatory secondary to chronic otitis media.

(**b**) Axial computed tomographic view of a right ear, showing an unusual image of a sclerotic TTF (tensor tympani fold, *white arrow*) secondary to an invasive tympano-sclerosis. *Cog black arrow, M* malleus, *I,* incus

4.5.2 The Lower Unit of the Attic (Prussak's Space)

(Figs. 4.13, 4.14, and 4.21)

In 1867, Prussak described a superior pouch of the tympanic membrane located between Shrap-nell's membrane and the neck of malleus and distinct from the anterior and posterior pouches of von Tröltsch. Later this superior pouch was renamed Prussak's space [40].

The Prussak's space is formed from the posterior pouch of von Tröltsch as a prolonga-tion of either a low portion or a high portion of the superior saccus, replacing the mesenchy-mal tissue between the neck of the malleus and Shrapnell's membrane [2]. The aeration pathway remains the same as the route of ori-gin which is the posterior pouch of von Tröltsch.

The Prussak's space is situated inferior to the tympanic diaphragm and represents the lower unit of the attic. Laterally, the Prussak's space extends superior to the roof of the external audi-tory canal by 0.4 mm and attains its largest cross section of 2.6 mm at the level of the roof of the external ear canal [4]. It presents the following limits:

- *The roof* is the lateral malleal fold which is a low portion of the tympanic diaphragm.

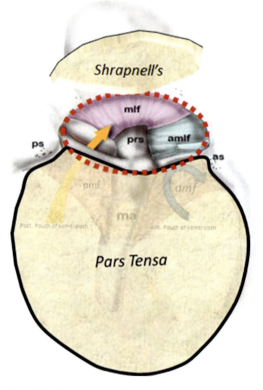

Fig. 4.21 Lateral view of the Prussak's space (*prs*) after reflection of the Shrapnell's membrane. *mlf* lateral malleal fold, *amlf* anterior malleal ligamental fold, *ps* posterior tym-panic spine, *as* anterior tympanic spine. *Yellow arrow*, aera-tion of Prussak's space through the posterior pouch of von Tröltsch. Reproduced with modification from Marchioni [44, Fig. 1] (With kind permission from Springer Science and Business Media, Springer and the original publisher)

- *The floor* is formed by the neck of the malleus.
- *The anterior limit* is the anterior malleal fold.
- *The lateral wall* is formed by the pars flaccida and the lower edge of the outer attic wall, the scutum.
- *The posterior wall* is opened to the posterior pouch of von Tröltsch and then to the mesotympanum.

The Prussak's space ventilation route is independent of the upper unit of the attic. The Prussak's space is ventilated through the posterior pouch of von Tröltsch which is particularly rough and narrow, as compared to the tympanic isthmus that is wider and provides large ventilation of the upper unit of the attic [32] (Fig. 4.21).

Clinical Applications
**Prussak's Space Dysventilation
and Attical Cholesteatoma**
The possibility of closure of the posterior pouch of von Tröltsch following thick mucus secretion formation during chronic inflammatory otitis is high. This event may cause a selective dysventilation of Prussak's space and development of pars flaccida retraction pocket with adhesion to the malleus neck (Fig. 4.22). This event may take place without any involvement of the other compartments of the upper unit that are situated superior to the tympanic diaphragm [41].

Initially the sac of the retraction pocket remains small and superficial to the ossicles. However, continued retraction and keratin accumulation lead to enlargement of the sac and its expansion via pathways of least resistance.

The growth pathways of attical cholesteatoma could be one of the following (Fig. 4.23):

Pathway 1: The cholesteatoma progresses through the posterior pouch of von Tröltsch. The posterior tympano-malleolar fold directs this expansion towards the inferior incudal space. From there, cholesteatoma may extend medial to the long process of the incus and then, through the tympanic isthmus, into the medial attic (Fig. 4.24).

Pathway 2: The cholesteatoma progresses through a thin part of the lateral malleal fold directly to the upper unit of the attic and from there to the posterior attic, aditus, and then to the antrum (Fig. 4.25).

Pathway 3: The cholesteatoma progresses from the lateral malleal space to the anterior attic, anterior epitympanic recess, and then it extends downwards to invade the supratubal recess and the protympanum (Fig. 4.26).

It should be emphasized that the folds of the attic direct the spread of cholesteatoma, but they do not constitute effective barriers to retain its expansion [4].

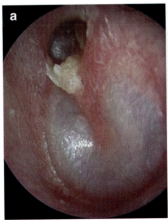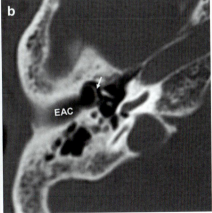

Fig. 4.22 (**a**) Attical cholesteatoma. (**b**) Transversal computed tomographic view of a right ear, showing a retraction pocket with its thickened capsule (*white arrow*) in the Prussak's space, extending anteriorly into the lateral attic. *EAC* external auditory canal

Fig. 4.23 Attical cholesteatoma growth pattern. From the Prussak's space cholesteatoma can extend through one of the following three tracts: (*1*) through the posterior pouch of von Tröltsch to the lower lateral attic (inferior incudal space, *IIS*), (*2*) through a defect in the lateral malleal fold (*LMF*) to the lateral malleal space (*LMS*) and then to the superior incudal space (*SIS*), or (*3*) from the lateral malleal space through the superior malleal fold defect (*SMF*) to the anterior attic. *SIF* superior incudal fold, *PIL* posterior incudal ligament, *MIF* medial incudal fold, *M* malleus, *LP* lateral process of malleus, *AMLF* anterior malleal ligamental fold

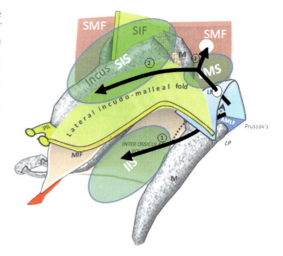

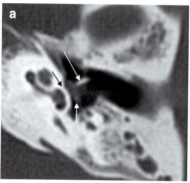
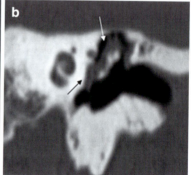

Fig. 4.24 Transversal (**a**) and coronal (**b**) computed tomographic view of a left ear with cholesteatoma growing according to the first pathway (Fig. 4.23). (**a**) Obliteration of the interossicular space between the malleus handle (*long white arrow*) and the long process of the incus (*short white arrow*) reaching the promontory (*black arrow*). (**b**) Further growth of the cholesteatoma from the medial mesotympanum (*black arrow*) to the medial attic (*white arrow*) along the ossicular chain

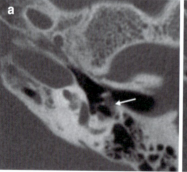
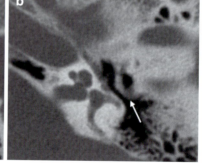

Fig. 4.25 Transversal computed tomographic view of a left ear showing a cholesteatoma growing from the Prussak's space according to the second pathway (Fig. 4.23). (**a**) Obliteration of the superior incudal space (*white arrow*). (**b**) On a more superior cut than (**a**), the obliteration shows a convex posterior contour (*white arrow*) due to the anatomical configuration of the lateral incudomalleal fold and the posterior incudal ligament

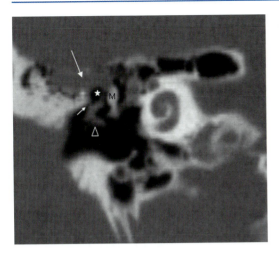

Fig. 4.26 Coronal computed tomographic view of a cholesteatoma in a right ear growing to the anterior epitympanum (*long arrow*) according to the third pathway (Fig. 4.23): retraction pocket from the Prussak's space (*), with amputation of the scutum (*short arrow*), detached keratine debris (*empty arrowhead*). *M* malleus

4.6 The Mesotympanum

The mesotympanum is the central and the biggest compartment of the middle ear cavity. However, it is the narrowest one; its depth is about 2 mm only. It is limited medially by the promontory and laterally by the pars tensa of the tympanic membrane. It is widely open anteriorly, inferiorly, and posteriorly to the protympanum, hypotympanum, and retrotympanum, retrospectively. Superiorly it is separated from the attic by the tympanic diaphragm.

The mesotympanum acts like a channel, allowing air coming from the Eustachian tube, to pass through the tympanic isthmus upward to provide aeration of the whole attic.

The lateral wall of the mesotympanum houses two important compartments:

4.6.1 Tympanic Membrane Compartments (Fig. 4.27)

4.6.1.1 Tympanic Membrane Pouches

- Anterior pouch of von Tröltsch: This pouch is situated between the anterior malleal fold and the pars tensa of the eardrum; it communicates with the supratubal recess and the protympanum [42].
- Posterior pouch of von Tröltsch: This pouch is situated between the posterior malleal fold and the pars tensa of the eardrum. The posterior pouch of von Tröltsch develops posteroinferiorly, and it opens in the most cranial portion of the mesotympanum [42]. It is the main route of ventilation of the Prussak's space.

Fig. 4.27 Schema of a right middle ear lateral wall compartments after removal of the pars tensa, showing the anterior pouch of von Tröltsch (*APV*) that is isolated from the Prussak's space (*blue arrow*) and the posterior pouch of von Tröltsch (*PPV*) that is in communication with the Prussak's space (*yellow arrow*). *as* anterior tympanic spine, *ps* posterior tympanic spine, *amf* anterior malleal fold, *pmf* posterior malleal fold, *ma* malleus handle

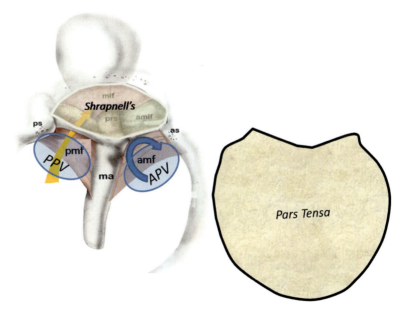

References

1. Proctor B. Embryology and anatomy of the Eustachian tube. Arch Otolaryngol. 1967;86:503–14.
2. Hammar JA. Studien ueber die Entwicklung des Vorderdarms und einiger angrenzender Organe. Arch Mikrosk Anat. 1902;59:471–628.
3. Proctor B. The development of the middle ear spaces and their surgical significance. J Laryngol Otol. 1964; 78:631–48.
4. Palva T, Johnsson LG. Epitympanic compartment surgical considerations: reevaluation. Am J Otol. 1995;16(4):505–13. Review. PubMed PMID: 8588652.
5. Onal K, Haastert RM, Grote JJ. Structural variations of supratubal recess: the anterior epitympanic space. Am J Otol. 1997;18:317–21. [PubMed].
6. Palva T, Ramsay H, Bohlurg J. Lateral and anterior view to tensor fold and supratubal recess. Am J Otol. 1998;19:405–14.
7. Giddings NA, Brackmann DE, Kwartler JA. Transcanal infracochlear approach to the petrous apex. Otolaryngol Head Neck Surg. 1991;104(1):29–36.
8. Mosnier I, Wu H, Chelly H, Cyna-Gorse F, Sterkers O. [Infralabyrinthine approach for cholesterol granuloma of the petrous apex]. Ann Otolaryngol Chir Cervicofac. 2000;117(3):174–82.
9. Ghorayeb BY, Jahrsdoerfer RA. Subcochlear approach for cholesterol granulomas of the inferior petrous apex. Otolaryngol Head Neck Surg. 1990;103(1):60–5.
10. Roland Jr JT, Hoffman RA, Miller PJ, Cohen NL. Retrofacial approach to the hypotympanum. Arch Otolaryngol Head Neck Surg. 1995;121(2):233–6.
11. Calli C, Pinar E, Oncel S, Tatar B, Tuncbilek MA. Measurements of the facial recess anatomy: implications for sparing the facial nerve and chorda tympani during posterior tympanotomy. Ear Nose Throat J. 2010;89:490–4.
12. Dahm MC, Shepherd RK, Clark GM. The postnatal growth of the temporal bone and its implications for cochlear implantation in children. Acta Otolaryngol Suppl. 1993;505:4–27.
13. Eby TL, Nadol JB. Postnatal growth of the human temporal bone: implications for cochlear implants in children. Ann Otol Rhinol Laryngol. 1986; 95:356–64.
14. Eby TL. Development of the facial recess: implications for cochlear implantation. Laryngoscope. 1996;106:1–7.
15. Bielamowicz SA, Coker NJ, Jenkins HA, Igarashi M. Surgical dimensions of the facial recess in adults and children. Arch Otolaryngol Head Neck Surg. 1988; 114(5):534–7.
16. Dahm M, Seldon HL, Pyman BC, Clark GM. 3D reconstruction of the temporal bone in cochlear implant surgery. In: Yanagihara N, Suziki J, editors. Transplants and implants in otology II. Amsterdam: Kugler; 1992. p. 271–5.
17. Parlier-Cuau C, Champsaur P, Perrin E, Rabischong P, Lassau JP. High-resolution computed tomographic

18. Proctor B. Surgical anatomy of the posterior tympanum. Ann Otol Rhinol Laryngol. 1969;78(5):1026–40.
19. Young YS, Nadol Jr JB. Dimensions of the extended facial recess. Ann Otol Rhinol Laryngol. 1989;98(5 Pt 1):336–8.
20. Bettman RH, Appelman AM, van Olphen AF, Zonneveld FW, Huizing EH. Cochlear orientation and dimensions of the facial recess in cochlear implantation. ORL J Otorhinolaryngol Relat Spec. 2003;65(6):353–8.
21. Jansen C. Posterior tympanotomy: experiences and surgical details. Otolaryngol Clin North Am. 1972; 5(1):79–96.
22. Anson BJ, Donaldson JA. Surgical anatomy of the temporal bone and ear. 2nd ed. Philadelphia: Saunders; 1981.
23. Marchioni D, Molteni G, Presutti L. Endoscopic anatomy of the middle ear. Indian J Otolaryngol Head Neck Surg. 2011;63(2):101–13.
24. Holt JJ. Posterior sinus of the middle ear. Ann Otol Rhinol Laryngol. 2007;116(6):457–61.
25. Ozturan O, Bauer C, Miller C, et al. Dimensions of the sinus tympani and its surgical access via retrofacial approach. Ann Otol Rhinol Laryngol. 1996;105: 776–83.
26. Nitek S, Wysocki J, Niemczyk K, Ungier E. The anatomy of the tympanic sinus. Folia Morphol (Warsz). 2006;65(3):195–9.
27. Amjad AH, Starke JJ, Scheer AA. Tympanofacial recess in the human ear. Arch Otolaryngol. 1968;88(2): 131–7.
28. Donaldson JA, Anson BJ, Warpeha RL, et al. The surgical anatomy of the sinus tympani. Arch Otolaryngol. 1970;91:219–27.
29. Thomassin JM, Danvin BJ, Collin M. Endoscopic anatomy of the posterior tympanum. Rev Laryngol Otol Rhinol (Bord). 2008;129(4–5):239–43.
30. Thomassin JM, Korchia D, Doris JM. Endoscopic-guided otosurgery in the prevention of residual cholesteatomas. Laryngoscope. 1993;103:939–43.
31. Palva T, Ramsay H, Northrop C. Color atlas of the anatomy and pathology of the epitympanum. Basel: Karger; 2001.
32. Palva T, Ramsay H, Böhling T. Prussak's space revisited. Am J Otol. 1996;17(4):512–20. PubMed PMID: 8841695.
33. Savic D, Djeric D. Anatomical variations and relations of the medial and lateral portions of the attic and their surgical significance. J Laryngol Otol. 1987;101(11):1109–17.
34. Palva T, Johnsson LG, Ramsay H. Attic aeration in temporal bones from children with recurring otitis media: tympanostomy tubes did not cure disease in Prussak's space. Am J Otol. 2000;21:485–93.
35. Palva T, Ramsay H. Chronic inflammatory ear disease and cholesteatoma: creation of auxiliary attic aeration pathways by microdissection. Am J Otol. 1999; 20:145–51.

study of the retrotympanum. Anatomic correlations. Surg Radiol Anat. 1998;20(3):215–20.

36. Horn KL, Brackmann DE, Luxford WM, et al. The supratubal recess in cholesteatoma surgery. Ann Otol Rhinol Laryngol. 1986;95:12–5.

37. Mansour S, Nicolas K, Naim A, et al. Inflammatory chronic otitis media and the anterior epitympanic recess. J Otolaryngol. 2005;34:149–58.

38. Hoshino T. Surgical anatomy of the anterior epitympanic space. Arch Otolaryngol Head Neck Surg. 1988;114:1143–5.

39. Todd NW, Heindel NH, PerLee JH. Bony anatomy of the anterior epitympanic space. ORL J Otorhinolaryngol Relat Spec. 1994;56:146–53.

40. Prussak A. Zur Anatomie des menschlichen Trommelfells. Arch Ohrenheilkd. 1867;3:255–78.

41. Palva T, Ramsey H. Aeration of Prussak's space is independent of the supradiaphragmatic epitympanic compartment. Otol Neurotol. 2007;28:264–8.

42. Von Tröltsch A. Lehrbuch der Ohrenheilkunde mit Einschluss der anatomie des Ohres. 7th ed. Leipzig: FCW Vogel; 1881.

43. Mansour S et al. Chronic inflammatory otitis media and the anterior epitympanic recess. J Otolaryngol. 2005;34(3):149–59.

44. Marchioni D. Lateral endoscopic approach to epitympanic diaphragm and Prussak's space: a dissection study. Surg Radiol Anat. 2010;32(9):843–52.

The Mastoid

5

Contents

The term "mastoid" is derived from the Greek word *mastós*, meaning breast, in reference to the shape of this bone. The mastoid process projects from the base of the skull and is situated behind the external auditory meatus at the inferior part of the outer surface of the temporal bone.

The mastoid process houses several important structures such as the facial nerve, the sigmoid sinus, and the labyrinth; it neighbors the middle and the posterior cranial fossa. Therefore, a good knowledge of the mastoid process anatomy is essential to approach it surgically and to avoid pitfalls.

Furthermore, the mastoid process is the site of numerous air-filled cavities known as mastoid air cells which play an important role in middle ear aeration.

5.1 Embryology of the Mastoid

The mastoid process appears at the 29th week of gestation as a result of the fusion of the periosteal layers of the otic capsule and the tympanic process of the squamous bone (see Figs. 1.1 and 1.3).

At birth, the mastoid process is underdeveloped; it becomes prominent by the age of 2 years and continues to grow until the age of 6 years. The expansion of the mastoid process is an active phenomenon and is secondary to the pneumatization process taking place inside it.

The pneumatization is a process in which the mastoid process, initially containing bone marrow, is invaded by the expanding air filled sacci. Thereafter, the mastoid becomes the site of an air-containing cavity called the mastoid air cells. The residual dense bone which did not pneumatize forms the septations between the mastoid air cells [1–12].

5.1.1   Embryology of the Mastoid Antrum

The antrum, which is the biggest of all mastoid air cells, starts its development between the 22nd and the 24th week of fetal life. It reaches its adult size on the 35th week [1, 13, 14].

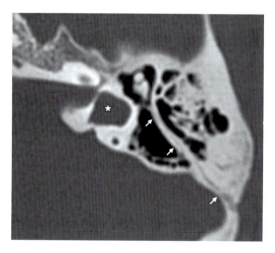

Fig. 5.1 Transversal computed tomography view of a left ear. Thin hyperlucent line (*white arrows*) along the fusion zone between the squamous and petrosal part of the mastoid, resulting in a bilamellar Korner's septum. Developmental arrest of the vestibule (*)

The antrum develops at the center of the mastoid process on both sides of the petrosquamous fissure. The medial part of the antrum, the petrous part, develops from the saccus medius and the lateral part, the squamous part, develops from the saccus superior (Figs. 4.2 and 4.3) (see Chap. 4). The fusion plane between the petrous part and the squamous part gives the petrosquamous fissure. Failure of complete fusion between the two sacci leads to a septation of the mastoid antrum by a bony partition called the Korner's septum [15] (Fig. 5.1).

The antrum is well developed at birth and has a mean surface of 1 cm^2 [16]. The size of the antrum does not change after birth; however, it undergoes medial displacement because of the growth of the mastoid process. The mastoid process continues to grow until puberty and even beyond.

5.1.2   Postnatal Mastoid Pneumatization

At birth, the mastoid process contains only the antrum. After birth, mastoid air cells develop as an outgrowth of the antrum; epithelial air tracts bud from the antrum and extend to the adjacent areas of the temporal bone to form the mastoid air cells (Fig. 5.2). This extension is facilitated by the differentiation of bone marrow into loose mesenchyme. This process is called mastoid pneumatization.

5.1.2.1   The Tracts of Pneumatization
Mastoid pneumatization proceeds through several well-established tracts. These tracts of pneumati-

Fig. 5.2 Transversal computed tomography of right ears: (**a**) in a newborn, showing the antrum (*) as the only air cell at this age; (**b**) in a child of 2 years old, showing advanced mastoid pneumatization medial and inferior to the antrum (*arrows*)

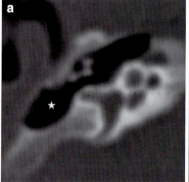
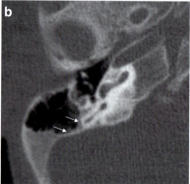

zation vary considerably. The main tracts of pneumatization are the following:

The Posterosuperior Cell Tract

The posterosuperior tract extends medially from the antrum at the junction of the posterior and middle fossa dural plates and above the superior semicircular canal and the internal auditory canal. It pneumatizes the medial pyramid of the temporal bone.

The Posteromedial Cell Tract (Superior Retrolabyrinthine)

The posteromedial tract extends medially through the antrum, parallel and inferior to the posterosuperior tract, to pneumatize the medial pyramid.

The Subarcuate Cell Tract (Translabyrinthine)

The subarcuate tract is situated more medially. It arises from the mastoid antrum and extends anteromedially passing below the superior semicircular canal; it pneumatizes the petrous apex.

The Perilabyrinthine Cell Tract

The perilabyrinthine cell tract arises from the antrum and pneumatizes the labyrinthine area. It is divided into the supralabyrinthine and the infralabyrinthine tracts. It can extend to the petrous apex.

The Peritubal Tract

This tract arises from the mastoid antrum and pneumatizes the tubal and peritubal area passing inferior to the labyrinth.

5.1.2.2 Mastoid Pneumatization Phases

The pneumatization of the mastoid begins at the 33rd week of gestation and ceases around puberty [1, 2, 17]. The last air cells to develop are the cells of the petrous apex. These air cells are present in about 35–40 % of adult temporal bones [2, 18, 19].

From birth until puberty, three phases of mastoid pneumatization are distinguishable:

- Phase I (0–1 year): The antrum is of adult size at birth and has a mean surface of 1 cm^2 (Fig. 5.2). During the first year of life, there is a rapid development of mastoid air cells. These new mastoid air cells add 3 cm^2 to the whole surface of mastoid air cell system, resulting in a total surface of 4 cm^2 at the age of 1 year.

  In the same time the mastoid process increases 1 cm in length and width and 0.5 cm in depth.

- Phase II (1–6 years): during this phase, mastoid pneumatization follows a linear pattern adding about 1 cm^2 per year. At the age of 2 years, the mastoid tip covers the emergence of the facial nerve at the stylomastoid foramen. The mastoid process growth increases then by about 0.5 cm per year in length and width and 0.25 cm per year in depth (Fig. 5.2).

- Phase III (6 years–puberty): during this phase the pneumatization process is very slow. It continues until puberty when the aerated mastoid process reaches its adult size. The mean adult mastoid air cells surface is about 12 cm^2 [2, 16].

Postnatal mastoid pneumatization displays considerable variation and this is related to several factors including heredity, environment, infections, and Eustachian tube function. A controversy exists concerning the relationship between the degree of mastoid pneumatization and the development of middle ear diseases. There are two theories:

1. Environmental theory: according to this theory, middle ear diseases presenting early in childhood are the cause of the failure of the pneumatization process to develop in infants and children [4–7, 20–22].

2. Genetic theory: this theory relates the extent of pneumatization to genetic factors, where an inherited reduced pneumatization predisposes the children to otitis media [2, 8–10].

The mastoid process is underdeveloped at birth. This situation leaves the facial nerve relatively superficial and unprotected where it emerges from the stylomastoid foramen. During difficult delivery, the use of forceps may damage the facial nerve by compression at this level. At the age of 2 years, as the air cells develop, the lateral part of the mastoid process grows downwards and forward to form the mastoid tip, which covers the stylomastoid foramen and offers progressively a better protection to the emerging facial nerve.

5.2   Mastoid Process Anatomy

The adult mastoid process is cone shaped and is slightly oblique forward and downwards. Its anterior border is rounded and vertical. Its posterior border is inclined about 45° downwards and forward. Behind the superior part of the mastoid process, the mastoid foramen is situated where the mastoid emissary vein passes.

The squamous bone forms the anterosuperior portion of the mastoid process. The petrous bone forms its postero-inferior part. The junction of the two parts forms the petrosquamous suture. The petrosquamous suture runs vertically from the superior border of the mastoid process to join its antero-inferior border just above the mastoid tip (Fig. 5.3).

The mastoid process serves as a point of attachment for several muscles like the splenius capitis, the longissimus capitis, the digastric, and the sternocleidomastoid muscles. The mastoid process is larger in men because they require larger points of attachment for their bigger muscles. The sternocleidomastoid muscle inserts to the outer surface of the mastoid tip. The posterior belly of digastric muscle inserts on the digastric groove situated on the inner surface of the mastoid tip. The digastric groove is an infallible guide to point the facial nerve emergence from the stylomastoid foramen at the anterior end of the groove.

5.2.1   Surface Landmarks of the Mastoid Process

Along the lateral surface of the mastoid process, we distinguish several important surgical landmarks:

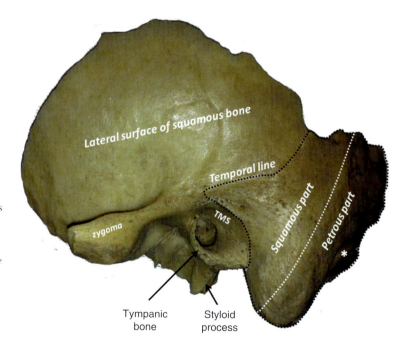

Fig. 5.3 Lateral surface of a left temporal bone, showing the mastoid process (*black dotted line*) formed from a squamous part and a petrous part, joined by the petrosquamous suture (*white dotted line*). The mastoid process is attached to the tympanic bone by the tympanomastoid suture (*TMS*); * digastric notch

Lateral surface of squamous bone

Temporal line

zygoma

TMS

Squamous part

Petrous part

Tympanic bone

Styloid process

5.2.1.1 Temporal Line

The temporal line is a horizontal ridge situated at the upper limit of the mastoid process. It extends behind the posterior root of the zygomatic process and marks the inferior margins of the insertion of the temporal muscle (Fig. 5.3). The temporal line may be a prominent sharp edge or a broad prominence. It may be absent [23].

> **Surgical Pearl**
> It is widely accepted that the temporal line is indicative of the inferior level of the middle fossa dura. Hence, during mastoidectomy, it is always recommended to drill along, not above, the temporal line in order to avoid inadvertent injury to the dura [24].
> Cadaveric studies found that the temporal line is located about 5 mm inferior to the middle fossa dura [25]. This may suggest that the drilling could start even at 5 mm above the temporal line without danger to the dura in order to increase the surgical exposure of the mastoid antrum.
> The distance between the temporal line and the middle fossa dura tends to be bigger in temporal bones with an absent Henle's spine [25, 26]. In cases where the temporal line is absent, the Henle's spine could be used as an anatomic criterion to presume the level of the middle fossa dura.

5.2.1.2 Henle's Spine

Henle's spine is a prominent bony plate seen on the outer surface of the mastoid process. It is situated behind and above the posterosuperior quadrant of the external auditory meatus and below the origin of the temporal line [26]. This lamella is incurved nearly concentrically to the circumference of the meatus and its upper extremity is more anterior than its inferior one (Fig. 5.4). Henle's spine could be small and smooth or sharp and long. It is absent in about 6 % of temporal bones [27, 28]. It serves as a point of attachment to the ligaments fixing the cartilaginous parts of the external acoustic meatus.

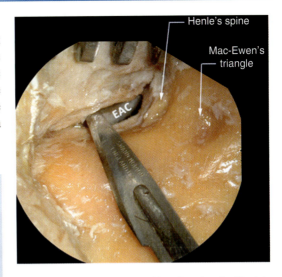

Fig. 5.4 Left cadaveric mastoid surface showing Henle's spine and Mac-Ewen's triangle. *EAC* external auditory canal

> **Surgical Pearl**
> Henle's spine is an excellent landmark during mastoidectomy because it indicates the region of the deeply located aditus ad antrum. In addition it may serve as a landmark for middle fossa dura when the temporal line is absent; the dura is situated about 1 cm superior to Henle's spine [25].

5.2.1.3 Mac-Ewen's Triangle

The suprameatal triangle or "Mac-Ewen's triangle" is a depression on the lateral surface of the mastoid process. It is located just between the anterior end of the temporal line, Henle's spine, and the posterosuperior quadrant of the external acoustic meatus (Fig. 5.4).

> **Surgical Pearl**
> Mac-Ewen's triangle is a useful anatomic landmark for the surgical access to the antrum; the mastoid antrum lies about 12–15 mm deeper to this triangle. This triangle is absent in 10 % of the population [29–32].

Fig. 5.5 Transverse cut of a left cadaveric temporal bone showing the antrum at the level of the aditus ad antrum (*). *PFP* posterior fossa plat, *EAC* external auditory canal, *1* attic outer wall, *2* anterior wall of the EAC, *3* posterior wall of the EAC, *C* cochlea, *sscc* superior semicircular canal, *m* malleus, *VII* facial nerve, *IC* internal carotid artery, *ET* Eustachian tube, *ma* middle meningeal artery, *TMJ* temporomandibular joint

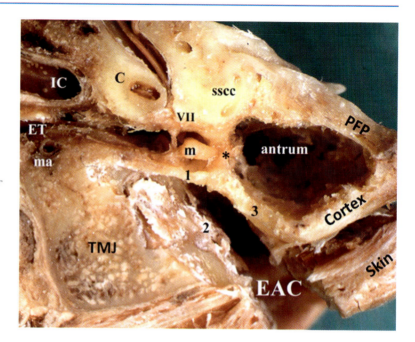

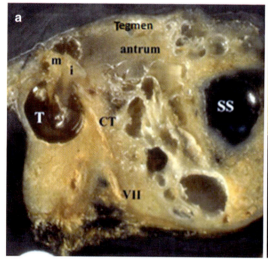
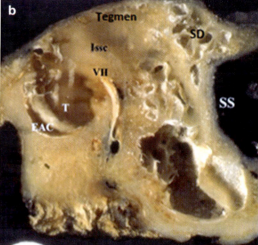

Fig. 5.6 Sagittal cuts through the temporal bone, showing in (**a**) the lateral wall of the antrum and in (**b**) the medial wall of the antrum containing the labyrinth. Notice that the antrum is posterosuperior to the tympanic cavity (*T*). The tegmen antrum slopes down as it goes anteriorly.

Sino-dural angle cells (*SD*) are located posterior to the antrum between the sigmoid sinus (*SS*) and the tegmen. The facial nerve VII is anteroinferior to the antrum. *EAC* external auditory canal, *m* malleus, *i* incus, *lssc* lateral semicircular cana, *CT* chorda tympani

5.2.2 Surgical Anatomy of the Mastoid Antrum

The mastoid antrum is the biggest mastoid air cell. It is of 10×10 mm in dimensions. It is located posterior to the external auditory canal and middle ear, inferior to the middle fossa dural plate, and anterior to the sigmoid sinus and the posterior fossa dural plate. The mastoid antrum communicates anteriorly with the attic through the aditus ad antrum (Figs. 5.5 and 5.6).

Fig. 5.7 A left mastoidectomy showing the antrum, with the lateral semicircular canal (*LSSC*) in its medial wall. Notice the relation between the Henle's spine (*S*) and the antrum: the antrum is always superior and posterior to the spine and the external auditory canal (*EAC*)

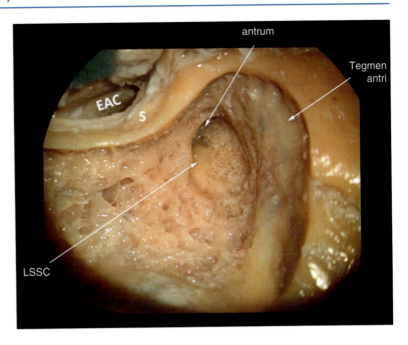

The depth of the mastoid antrum is a cardinal point in mastoid surgery. Despite the fact that the antrum reaches its adult size at birth, its medial displacement secondary to the pneumatization process renders its depth dependent of the age of the subject. Its depth varies also from person to person of the same age. In infants less than 1- year-old, the distance between the cortical bone and the antrum is only 2–4 mm (Fig. 5.2a). At 3 years old, the antrum is at 10 mm from the cortical bone, and in the adult, the antrum may be at 25 mm from the mastoid cortical bone [33].

5.2.2.1 Position of the Antrum in Relation to Surface Landmarks

In young children, the antrum is quickly reached by curetting the cortical bone. In adults, the antrum is situated below the supramastoid ridge, above and in front of the petrosquamous suture. Mac-Ewen's triangle is an important indicator of the antrum's area (compare Figs. 5.4 and 5.7).

The relation of the antrum and Henle's spine is age-dependent because the antrum has an inferior and posterior migration during the postnatal period. Near the age of 10 years, it is on the horizontal track designed by the Henle's spine; after this age, the antrum sets about 1 cm behind Henle's spine.

5.2.2.2 Deep Relationships of the Antrum

Several important structures must be considered while operating on the mastoid antrum; the most important are the horizontal semicircular canal, the facial nerve, the lateral sinus, the posterior fossa dural plate, and the tegmen antri. Knowing the anatomy of the antrum and its relation to these structures is essential to carry out a safe mastoid surgery.

The Horizontal Semicircular Canal and the Solid Triangle

Medially, the antrum is limited by the solid triangle of the mastoid, which is the bony angle formed by the three semicircular canals.

The horizontal semicircular canal is situated just behind the inner wall of the antrum. The canal is surrounded by a solid compact bony shell, which by itself offers a strong resistance to instruments. The distance from the tegmen antri to the lateral semicircular canal is about 6 mm [25].

The superior semicircular canal runs perpendicular to the lateral canal. It is about 2 mm more

Fig. 5.8 Cadaveric left mastoidectomy showing lateral semicircular canal (*LSCC*), the superior semicircular canal (*SSCC*), and the posterior semicircular canal (*PSCC*). Notice the relationship between the PSCC and the facial nerve (*VII*). Notice the Donaldson's line (the *black dotted line*) and the endolymphatic sac (*)

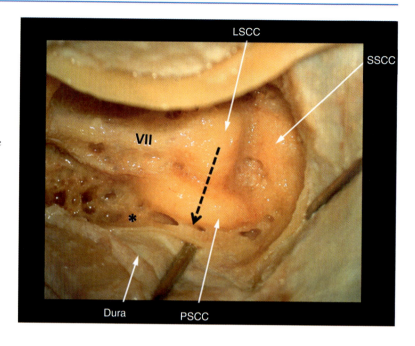

medially situated. Its anterior crus runs superiorly towards the tegmen tympani and then curves posteriorly to join the posterior semicircular canal forming the common crus. The posterior canal also runs perpendicular to the lateral canal. The superior half of the posterior canal is located superior to a line bisecting the lateral canal called Donaldson's line. The inferior half of the posterior canal runs inferiorly to the Donaldson's line and emerges deep to the vertical portion of the facial nerve to enter the vestibule (Fig. 5.8).

Surgical Application
Donaldson's Line
Donaldson's line is a straight line that runs in the axis of the horizontal semicircular canal and bisects the posterior semicircular canal. It is an important landmark for searching the endolymphatic sac (Fig. 5.8). The endolymphatic sac sits on the posterior fossa dura inferior to Donaldson's line and medial to the labyrinth. Surgical exposure of the endolymphatic sac is carried out through the retrofacial air cells tract in the area bounded: anteriorly by the mastoid segment of the facial nerve, posteriorly by the posterior fossa plate, superiorly by the posterior semicircular canal, and inferiorly by the jugular bulb.

The Petromastoid Canal
The petromastoid canal is a canal that runs from the posterior cranial fossa to the mastoid antrum; it is usually vestigeous and closed. It starts at the fossa subarcuata, situated on the posterior surface of the temporal bone superiorly and posteriorly in relation to the internal auditory canal. It traverses the temporal bone laterally underneath the superior semicircular canal and above the lateral semicircular canal to reach the mastoid antrum (Fig. 5.9). It establishes a potential communication between the mastoid cavity and the endocranium. If it is patent, it may be a cause of recurrent meningitis.

The Mastoid Segment of the Facial Nerve
The vertical part of the Fallopian canal drops down in the anterior wall of the mastoid cavity in a plane almost parallel to the posterior wall of the external auditory canal. It passes through a compact lamina of bone known under the name of the arc-lied premastoid lamina.

In adults, the inferior part of the antrum neighbors the second genu of the facial nerve. The facial nerve must be recognized as it emerges from the tympanic cavity between the horizontal semicircular canal medial and the short process of the incus. The incudal process is always more than 2 mm lateral to the facial

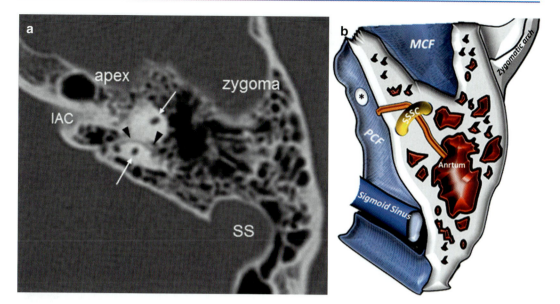

Fig. 5.9 (a) Transversal computed tomography of a left ear mastoid at the level of the petromastoid canal (*black arrowheads*) in between the two arms of the superior semicircular canal (*white arrows*). *SS* sigmoid sinus, *IAC* internal auditory canal. (**b**) Schema showing a right petromastoid canal taking origin from the posterior cranial fossa (*PCF*) anterosuperior to the internal auditory canal (***) and passing below the superior semicircular canal (*SSSC*) to the antrum. *MCF* middle cranial fossa

nerve and it is an important landmark to localize the facial nerve.

In children, the antrum is highly situated in relation to the facial nerve; therefore, the surgical approach to the antrum is of a low risk for an eventual facial injury.

The distance from the vertical segment of the facial nerve to the posterior fossa dura ranges from 5 to 10 mm [3]. The distance between the mastoid segment of the facial nerve canal and the sigmoid sinus is highly variable; it is around 4 mm [34].

The distance between the facial nerve and the tympanic membrane annulus is about 2–3 mm.

The lower one-third of the mastoid segment of the facial nerve is in close proximity to the digastric ridge where the nerve is always medial and anterior to this structure. The digastric ridge represents a landmark for the facial nerve identification. At this level, the sigmoid sinus passes medially to the facial nerve (Fig. 5.10). In a poorly pneumatized temporal bone, the digastric ridge may be difficult to identify.

The facial nerve exits the Fallopian canal via the stylomastoid foramen. The mean depth of the facial nerve from the mastoid cortex at the stylomastoid foramen is 13 mm.

The Sigmoid Sinus

The sigmoid sinus is a continuation of the transverse sinus. It passes through the mastoid process in an anteroinferior direction to join the jugular bulb, forming a curvature with an anterior angle. The posterosuperior part of the sigmoid sinus is the most superficial part; from there, the sinus lays gradually deeper in the mastoid process. Inferiorly, at the level of the mastoid tip, it passes medial to the digastric ridge and the facial nerve to join the jugular bulb (Fig. 5.11).

At the junction with the jugular bulb, the sigmoid sinus receives the inferior petrosal sinus, which courses along the inferior portion of the posterior surface of the petrous pyramid. The superior petrosal sinus enters the sigmoid sinus at its junction with the transverse sinus. Both the superior and the inferior petrosal sinuses are connected to the cavernous sinus. The inferior petrosal sinus is also connected to the basilar plexus (Fig. 5.12).

The position of the sigmoid sinus with respect to the external auditory canal is variable. The distance from the sigmoid sinus to the posterior external auditory canal ranges from 10 to 20 mm [34]. This distance is dependent on the degree of the mastoid pneumatization. The sigmoid sinus could be very anterior in poorly pneumatized

Fig. 5.10 (**a**) Microscopic view showing posterior tympanotomy and the relationship between the second genu, the incus, and the lateral semicircular canal (*LSCC*). (**b**) View of the mastoid tip showing the relationship between the digastric ridge and the facial nerve

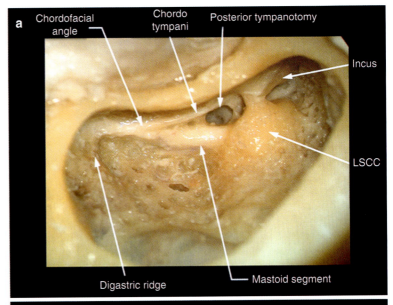

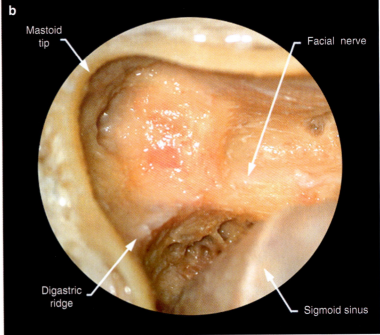

Fig. 5.11 Cadaveric left large mastoidectomy with skeletonization of the sigmoid sinus (*SS*). *MCF* middle cranial fossa

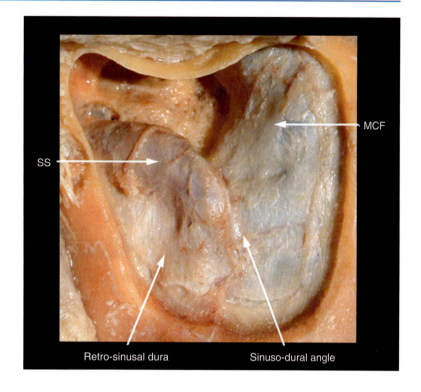

Fig. 5.12 Schema showing right sigmoid sinus and its connection with the cavernous sinus through the superior and inferior petrosal sinuses. *JB* jugular bulb

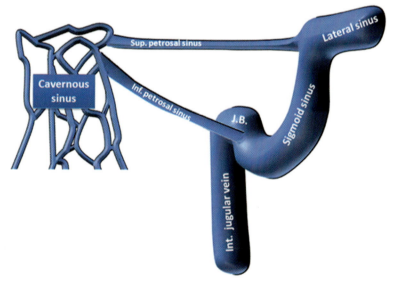

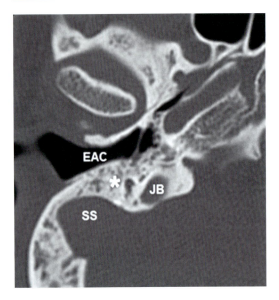

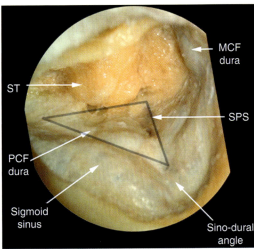

Fig. 5.14 Cadaveric large mastoidectomy showing the middle cranial fossa (*MCF*) and posterior cranial fossa (*PCF*) dura, the sino-dural angle, and the imaginary Trautman's triangle (*black lined triangle*). ST solid triangle, *SPS* superior petrosal sinus

Fig. 5.13 Transversal computed tomographic view of a sclerotic mastoid (*) of a right ear; the sigmoid sinus (*SS*) is very anterior and lateralized. *JB* jugular bulb, *EAC* external auditory canal

bones (Fig. 5.13). In a well-pneumatized mastoid process, the lateral aspect of the sigmoid sinus could be covered by mastoid air cells (Fig. 5.20).

> **Surgical Implication**
> The most common anatomic variant of the sigmoid sinus is its anterior displacement. This situation can obscure the view of the mastoid structures and pathology and eventually require a decompression to improve access to the needed structures (Fig. 5.13). Decompression is accomplished by removing bone around the sinus itself leaving a bony island plate that can be pressed down on the sinus without significant risk of tearing the sinus.
>
> Also bipolar cauterization of the sinus wall makes the sinus shrink and secondarily increase the space for a comfortable surgical approach.

The Posterior Fossa Dural Plate

The posterior fossa dural plate is a thin plate of bone that separates the mastoid antrum and

mastoid air cells from the posterior cranial fossa. It is demarcated by the superior petrosal sinus superiorly, by the sigmoid sinus latero-inferiorly, and by the posterior semicircular canal medially (Fig. 5.14).

The Tegmen Antri

The tegmen antri is the part of the tegmen lying above the mastoid antrum. It separates the antrum from the overlying middle fossa dura and the temporal lobe (see Sect. 2.4.2.2).

The Trautman's Triangle

The Trautman's triangle is an imaginary triangle bounded by the tegmen, the superior petrosal sinus, the sigmoid sinus, and the bony labyrinth (Fig. 5.14). Most of the posterior fossa dura is included in Trautman's triangle. In well-pneumatized temporal bones, the distance between the sigmoid sinus and the labyrinth may measure up to 10 mm. This distance may be much smaller. Exposure of Trautman's triangle is essential for the most neurosurgical approaches through the temporal bone. The access from the mastoid cavity to the posterior cranial fossa is gained by traversing this triangle.

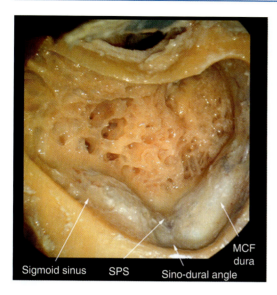

Sigmoid sinus   SPS   Sino-dural angle

MCF dura

Fig. 5.15 Left mastoidectomy, showing the sino-dural angle. *SPS* superior petrosal sinus, *MCF* middle cranial fossa

The Sino-dural Angle (The Citelli Angle)

The citelli angle is the angle between the middle fossa and the posterior fossa dural plates (Fig. 5.15). In a well-pneumatized mastoid, this angle is occupied by many small air cells, called Citelli cells. These cells must be completely exenterated during mastoidectomy for chronic suppurative otitis media; otherwise, persistent infection in these cells may lead to recurrence of the pathology. In certain cases drilling deep enough down into the angle to expose the superior petrosal sinus is mandatory in order to exenterate all these cells.

The Korner's Septum

The Korner's septum is a dense bony plate present inside the mastoid process. It is a persistent plate of bone in the plane of fusion of the two primordia of the mastoid antrum: the saccus medius and the saccus superior (see Sect. 4.1). This septum divides the mastoid process into a superficial squamous portion and a deep petrous portion. The Korner's septum extends from the posterior wall of the external auditory canal; it disperses in the air cells close to the middle fossa plate, the sino-dural angle, and the sigmoid sinus plate; it then runs inferiorly lateral to the facial canal as it proceeds to the mastoid tip.

> **Surgical Implication**
> During mastoid surgery, a well-developed Korner's septum may be mistaken for the medial wall of the antrum. If it is not recognized, the deep part of the antrum would not be exposed. A preoperative high-resolution CT scan of the temporal bone may demonstrate the presence of this septum (Fig. 5.1).

5.2.3 The Aditus Ad Antrum

The mastoid antrum communicates anteriorly with the attic of the middle ear through a narrow pathway called the aditus ad antrum.

The aditus ad antrum is a short and restricted bony canal situated at the posterior prolongation of the attic. It has a triangular shape with dimensions of $4 \times 4 \times 4$ mm height, length, and width. In adults, the aditus is present in the upper part of the anterior wall of the mastoid antrum. However, in newborns and infants, it is present in the middle part of this wall. This is because of the postnatal inferior migration of the mastoid antrum.

The aditus is bounded:
- *Superiorly* by the tegmen.
- *Medially* and *inferiorly* by the lateral semicircular canal; medial to the later is the second genu of the facial nerve.
- *Laterally* by the scutum.

At the level of the aditus, the lateral semicircular canal, the short process of the incus, and the second genu of the facial nerve are all closely related. The lateral semicircular canal is seen as a solid whitish bony prominence positioned from anterosuperior to posteroinferior at approximately 30° angle from the aditus. The second genu of the facial nerve is just inferior and medial to the lateral semicircular canal (Figs. 5.16 and 5.17).

5.2.4 The Mastoid Air Cells

The mastoid air cell system is categorized according to the various regions of the temporal bone. These air cells include:

Fig. 5.16 Left mastoidectomy showing the aditus ad antrum (*imaginary triangle*)

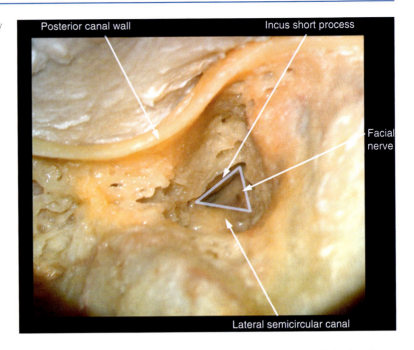

Posterior canal wall   Incus short process   Facial nerve   Lateral semicircular canal

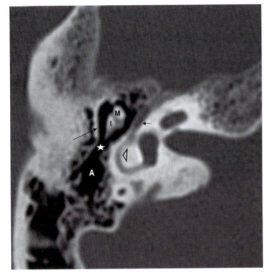

Fig. 5.17 Transversal computed tomography of a right ear showing the aditus ad antrum (*), connecting the antrum (*A*) to the epitympanum. Incus (*I*), malleus (*M*), scutum (*long arrow*), lateral semicircular canal (*empty arrowhead*), tympanic segment of the facial nerve (*short arrow*)

5.2.4.1 Squamomastoid Cells

These air cells are limited to the mastoid process itself and are subdivided into:

- *The antrum.*

- *The central mastoid tract,* which is the direct extension of the antrum inferiorly.
- *The peripheral mastoid area* arising from the antrum. The peripheral tract is further subdivided into tegmental cells above the external auditory canal, posterosuperior cells (sinodural angle), posteroinferior sinusal cells (around the sigmoid sinus), facial cells (around the mastoid portion of the facial nerve), and mastoid tip cells, which are divided into medial and lateral groups by the digastric ridge. Depending on their extension in regard to the sigmoid sinus, the mastoid cells are classified into presinusoidal, sinusoidal, and postsinusoidal mastoid cells.

5.2.4.2 Petrous Cells

The petrous cells are subdivided into perilabyrinthine cells and apical cells (Figs. 5.18 and 5.19).

Perilabyrinthine Cells

These are the air cells surrounding the labyrinth; they include the supralabyrinthine cells superior to the labyrinth and infralabyrinthine cells inferior to the labyrinth.

The supralabyrinthine cells are subdivided to posterosuperior, posteromedial, and subarcuate cells [1, 35]:

Fig. 5.18 Schematic drawing showing perilabyrinthine cells. *1* supralabyrinthine cells, *2* subarcuate cells, *3* posteromedial cells, *4* infralabyrinthine cells, * peritubal cells, *SS* sigmoid sinus, *IAC* internal auditory canal, *EAC* external auditory canal, *ET* Eustachian tube, *lscc* lateral semicircular canal, *pscc* posterior semicircular canal, *sscc* superior semicircular canal

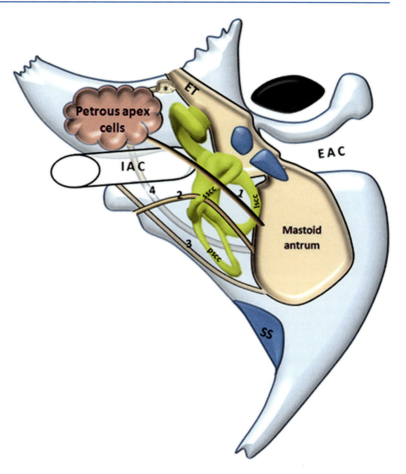

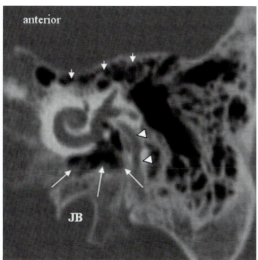

Fig. 5.19 Sagittal oblique computed tomographic reconstruction showing the supralabyrinthine air cells (*small arrows*) and the infralabyrinthine air cells (*long arrows*). Mastoid segment of the facial nerve (*arrow heads*). Jugular bulb (*JB*)

- *The posterosuperior cells*, arising from the antrum, are located around the superior semicircular canal and along the posterior surface of the petrous bone above the internal auditory canal.
- *The posteromedial cells* extend along the posterior surface of the petrous bone beneath the posterosuperior cells towards the posterior wall of the internal auditory canal [36].
- *The subarcuate cells* extend through the arch of the superior semicircular canal into the subarcuate fossa [1, 35].

Apical Cells

The apical cells are located medial to the internal auditory canal (IAC) and posteromedial to the carotid canal.

The degree of pneumatization of the petrous apex is variable and it is correlated with the extent of the mastoid cells [1, 35, 36]. The

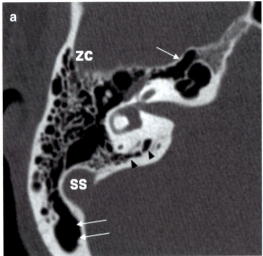 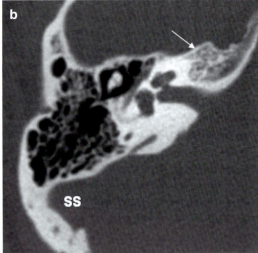

Fig. 5.20 Computed tomography of right ears. (**a**) Well-pneumatized petrous apex (*arrow*) with well-pneumatized postsinusoidal cells (*double arrows*), posteromedial retrolabyrinthine cells (*arrowheads*), zygomatic cells (*ZC*). (**b**) Diploic petrous apex (*arrow*); *SS* sigmoid sinus

petrous apex is usually occupied by a soft bone marrow and contains no air cells, so defined as diploic petrous apex. However, 30 % of patients have a petrous apex which contains air cells (pneumatized petrous apex) (Fig. 5.20) [18, 36]. The apical cells communicate with the perilabyrinthine cells laterally and with the peritubal cells anteriorly.

> **Clinical Implication**
> A communication between the mastoid antrum and the petrous apex exists through the perilabyrinthine cells (Figs. 5.18 and 5.20). The spread of an ear infection can involve the air cells around the petrous apex leading to osteomyelitis of the petrous apex, "petrous apicitis." Inflammation of this region may involve the sixth cranial nerve at the Dorello's canal and the fifth cranial nerve in the Meckel's cave giving symptoms of Gradenigo syndrome with the triad of a discharging ear, retro-orbital pain due to the involvement of trigeminal ganglion, and diplopia (see Fig. 1.14).

5.2.4.3 Accessory Air Cells

These cells include zygomatic, occipital, squamous, and styloid air cells (Fig. 5.20).

5.2.5 Mastoid Air Cell System Volume

The mastoid air cell system is covered with a vascularized cuboidal epithelium. The contact between the blood vessels and the basement membrane of this epithelium is rather close resembling that of the alveoli where extensive gaseous exchange takes place.

In addition, the mastoid air cell system serves as a reservoir of air and a buffer system to replace air in the middle ear cavity temporarily in case of Eustachian tube dysfunction.

The mean volume of air in the mastoid air cell system could be of about 5–8 ml. CT scan evaluation of the temporal bone is considered to be the best modality to assess the mastoid air cell system and the type of pneumatization (Fig. 5.21).

The pneumatization of the mastoid air cell system can be divided into three types:
1. Sclerotic mastoid – pneumatization is absent.
2. Diploic mastoid – pneumatization is partial.
3. Pneumatic mastoid – full and complete pneumatization.

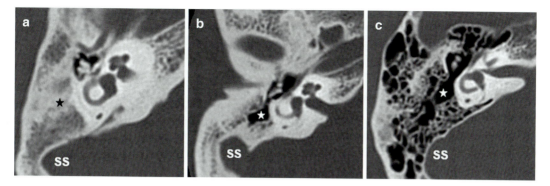

Fig. 5.21 Transversal computed tomographic views on right ears. (**a**) Completely sclerotic mastoid, even the antrum (*) is sclerotic; (**b**) small antrum (*) in diploic mastoid; (**c**) well-pneumatized mastoid and antrum (*). *SS* sigmoid sinus

References

1. Allam AF. Pneumatization of the temporal bone. Ann Otol Rhinol Laryngol. 1969;78:48–64.
2. Diamant M. Otitis and pneumatization of the mastoid bone. Acta Otolaryngol (Suppl) (Stockh). 1940;41:1–149.
3. Wittmaack K. Über die normale und Pathologische Pneumatization des Schlafenbeins einschiesslich ihrer Beziehungen zu der Mittelohrerkrankungen. Jena: Fischer; 1918. p. 1–64.
4. Gans H, Wlodyka J. Mastoid pneumatization in chronic otitis media. Acta Otolaryngol. 1966;33:343–6.
5. Palva T, Palva A. Size of the human mastoid air cell system. Acta Otolaryngol. 1966;62:237–51.
6. Hug JE, Pfaltz CR. Temporal bone pneumatization. A planimetric study. Arch Otorhinolaryngol. 1981;233:145–56.
7. Tos M. Mastoid pneumatization. A critical analysis of the hereditary theory. Acta Otolaryngol. 1982;94:73–80.
8. Ueda T, Eguchi S. Distribution of pneumatization of the temporal bone in chronic otitis media seen during the age of antibiotic therapy. J Otol Rhinol Laryngol (Japan). 1962;64:1539–42.
9. Schulter-Ellis F. Population differences in cellularity of the mastoid process. Acta Otolaryngol. 1979;87:461.
10. Sade J, Hadas E. Prognostic evaluation of secretory otitis media as a function of mastoidal pneumatization. Arch Otorhinolaryngol. 1979;225:39–44.
11. Holmquist J. Aeration in chronic otitis media. Clin Otolaryngol. 1978;3:278–84.
12. Sade J. The correlation of middle ear aeration with mastoid pneumatization. Eur Arch Otorhinolaryngol. 1992;249:301–4.
13. Bast TH, Forester HB. Origin and distribution of air cells in the temporal bone. Arch Otorhinolaryngol. 1939;30:183–205.
14. Bast TH, Anson BJ. The temporal bone and the ear. Springfield: Charles C Thomas; 1949. p. 162–291.
15. Virapongse C, Kirschrer JC, Sasaki C, et al. Computed tomography of Koerner's septum and the petrosquamosal suture. Arch Otolaryngol Head Neck Surg. 1986;112:81–7.
16. Cinamon U. The growth rate and size of the mastoid air cell system and mastoid bone: a review and reference. Eur Arch Otorhinolaryngol. 2009;266(6):781–6.
17. Rubensohn G. Mastoid pneumatization in children at various ages. Acta Otolaryngol (Stockh). 1965;60:11–4.
18. Virapongse C, Sarwar M, Bhimani S, Sasaki C, Shapiro R. Computed tomography of temporal bone pneumatization: 1 normal pattern and morphology. AJR Am J Roentgenol. 1985;145:473–81.
19. Hentona H, Ohkubo J, Tsutsumi T, Tanaka H, Komatsuzaki A. Pneumatization of the petrous apex. Nippon Jibiinkoka Gakkai Kaiho. 1994;97:450–6.
20. Tumarkin A. On the nature and significance of hypocellularity of mastoid. J Laryngol Otol. 1959;73:34–44.
21. Tumarkin A. On the nature and vicissitudes of the accessory air spaces of the middle ear. J Laryngol Otol. 1957;71:210–48.
22. Kolihova E, Abraham J, Blahova O. Rezidivierende Mittelohrentzündung im frühen Kindesalter und ihr Einfluss an die Zellsystementwicklung des Schlafenbeins. Radiologie. 1966;12:62–5.
23. Tos M. Manual of middle ear surgery, Mastoid surgery and reconstructive procedures, vol. 2. Stuttgart: Thieme; 1995.
24. Sanna M, Saleh E, Taibah A, Russo A. Atlas of temporal bone. 1st ed. Stuttgart: Thieme; 1995.
25. Aslan A, Mutlu C, Celik O, Govsa F, Ozgur T, Egrilmez M. Surgical implications of anatomical landmarks on the lateral surface of the mastoid bone. Surg Radiol Anat. 2004;26(4):263–7. Epub 2004 Jun 17.
26. Williams PL, Bannister LH, Berry MM, Collins P, Dyson M, Dussek JE, et al., editors. Gray's anatomy: the

anatomical basis of medicine and surgery. 38th ed. London: Churchill Livingstone; 1995. p. 56.

27. Anson B, Donaldson JA. Surgical anatomy of the temporal bone. 4th ed. New York: Raven; 1992.

28. Peker TV, Pelin C, Turgut HB, Anil A, Sevim A. Various types of suprameatal spines and depressions in the human temporal bone. Eur Arch Otorhinolaryngol. 1998;255:391–5.

29. Williams PL, Warwick R, Dyson M, Bannister LH. Gray's anatomy. 37th ed. Edinburg: ELBS with Churchill Livingstone; 1993.

30. Berkovitz BKB, Moxham BJ. A textbook of head and neck anatomy. London: Wolfe Medical; 1988.

31. Akabori E. Crania nipponica recentia. Analytical inquiries into the non-metric variations in the Japanese skull. Jpn J Med Sci I Anat. 1933;4:61–318, 11.

32. Romanes GJ (1992). Cunningham's manual of practical anatomy, vol III. Head and neck and brain. London: Oxford University Press.

33. Schwartze A. Handbuch der Ohrenheilkllnde. Leipzig: Vogel; 1893.

34. Măru N, Cheiţă AC, Mogoantă CA, Prejoianu B. Intratemporal course of the facial nerve: morphological, topographic and morphometric features. Rom J Morphol Embryol. 2010;51(2):243–8.

35. Pellet W, Cannoni M, Pech A. Basic anatomy. In: Otoneurosurgery. Berlin: Springer; 1990. p. 5–72.

36. Yamakami I, Uchino Y, Kobayashi E, Yamaura A. Computed tomography evaluation of air cells in the petrous bone – relationship with postoperative cerebrospinal fluid rhinorrhea. Neurol Med Chir (Tokyo). 2003;43(7):334–8; discussion.

Facial Nerve

6

Contents

The facial nerve, or cranial nerve (CN VII), is the nerve of facial expression. Due to various developmental events, the trajectory of the facial nerve, from its origin in the brainstem to the muscles of the face, is tortuous and complex. The ingenious pathway of the facial nerve through the middle ear and mastoid adds to the complexity and refinement of middle ear microsurgery. Thus, a thorough knowledge of the facial nerve anatomy along with its multiple landmarks is essential for an accurate, safe, and effective surgical intervention in the middle ear.

A basic understanding of the developmental anatomy is necessary to anticipate the various anatomical situations encountered during ear surgery.

6.1   Facial Nerve Development

The development of the motor root of the facial nerve is independent of the development of the sensory root and the geniculate ganglion.

The facial nerve primordium is first recognized at the 4th week of gestation as a collection of cells at the vicinity of the auditory placode, which will generate the otocyst (Fig. 6.1). These cells are derived from neural crest cells and epibranchial microplacodes of the second branchial arch. Then, the facial nerve primordium extends to the primitive geniculate ganglion region as a narrow band; meanwhile, the acoustic nerve has reached the otocyst [1].

S. Mansour et al., *Comprehensive and Clinical Anatomy of the Middle Ear*,
DOI 10.1007/978-3-642-36967-4_6, © Springer-Verlag Berlin Heidelberg 2013

Fig. 6.1 Frontal (asymmetric) section of a head of a E9 mouse embryo. At the right side, we observe facial nerve fibers (*arrow*) in contact with the rhombencephalon (*Rh*). At the left side, rudiment of the geniculate ganglion is visible (*large arrow*) at the vicinity of the otocyst (*O*) and the anterior cardinal vein (*V*). *I* and *II*, first and second branchial arches

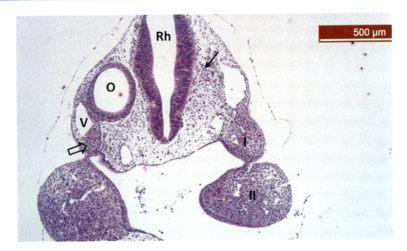

Fig. 6.2 Transverse section of a 13-mm human embryo, showing the close relationship of the facial nerve rudiment (*VII*) with the stapes (*S*) anlage, crossed by the stapedial artery (*SA*). Hematoxylin-eosin staining

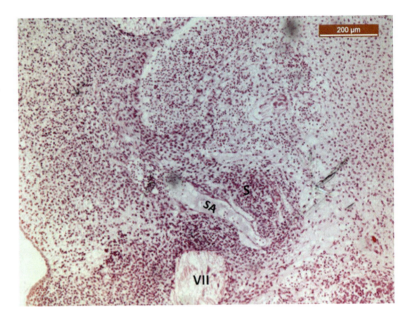

In the 5th week, the facial motor nucleus can be identified in the developing brainstem. Nerve fibers leave the nucleus and pass caudal to the region of the geniculate ganglion. These fibers bend dorsally to give the horizontal segment of the nerve which passes between the developing labyrinth and the upper end of the Reichert's cartilage. The upper end of the Reichert's cartilage will become the blastema of the stapes (Fig. 6.2). Finally the facial nerve bends vertically before passing into the substance of the second branchial arch, the laterohyale [1] (Fig. 6.3).

In the 5th week, the chorda tympani is the first branch of the facial nerve to appear. At this time, the chorda tympani nerve and the facial nerve trunk are of approximately equal size; this state could be encountered clinically in adult ears with major atresia [2]. The chorda tympani nerve (Fig. 6.3) dives into the mandibular arch to terminate in the same region as the lingual nerve ends and where the submandibular ganglion develops. The chorda tympani nerve primordium divides the mandibular ossicular blastema into malleus laterally and incus medially. By the 7th week, however, the chorda tympani nerve is smaller

Fig. 6.3 Frontal section in a 15.5-mm human embryo. The facial nerve rudiment (*VII*) is partially covered by the laterohyale (*L*), derived from the Reichert's cartilage, and crosses the stapes (*S*), itself traversed by the stapedial artery (*SA*). The anterior cardinal vein (*V*) is lateral to the nerve. Hematoxylin-eosin staining

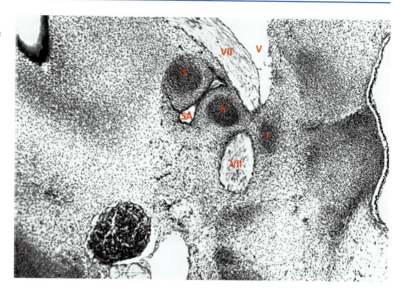

Fig. 6.4 A 15.5-mm human embryo, transverse section. Facial nerve is visible in close relationship with the Reichert's cartilage (*R*). Chorda tympani (*CT*) is more anterior, between first and second arches, in relationship with the malleus (*M*). *Ph* first pharyngeal pouch, *cleft* first branchial cleft. Hematoxylin-eosin staining

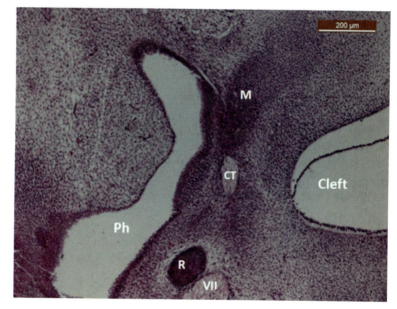

than the facial nerve and remains so until adulthood [2] (see Fig. 3.2).

In the 7th week, the sensory root of the facial nerve (nervus intermedius) arises from the geniculate ganglion and runs between the motor root of the facial nerve and the cochleovestibular nerve on its way to the brainstem. At the same time the greater petrosal nerve, which is the second branch of the facial nerve to appear, develops from the anterior aspect of the geniculate ganglion.

The mesenchyme around the facial nerve develops later into the facial nerve canal. The first cartilaginous anlage of the facial canal derives from the laterohyale (Figs. 6.3 and 6.4). The development of the contiguous structures, such as the stapes, the labyrinthine capsule, the mastoid bone, and the tympanic bone, will determine the ultimate trajectory of the facial nerve canal.

Originally, the facial nerve passes in a sulcus in the cartilaginous otic capsule; later this sulcus ossifies and becomes the bony canal of the facial nerve. The process of ossification has two centers:

- *An anterior center:* it develops at the apical cochlear ossification center by the end of the 20th week gestation.
- *A posterior center:* it arises at the pyramidal eminence by the 25th week of gestation [3].

Each ossification center emits two bony projections that ideally encircle progressively the entire length of the facial nerve. At term, about 80 % of the tympanic segment of the Fallopian canal is ossified; the ossification is almost completed around 3 months after birth. Facial nerve dehiscence is related to failure of complete fusion of these two ossification centers [3].

Surgical Pearl

At birth, the facial nerve exits the stylomastoid foramen on the lateral aspect of the skull, just inferior to the tympanic membrane and external ear canal. This makes the facial nerve vulnerable to traumatic injury during difficult delivery. In the second year of life, the growing mastoid process pushes the stylomastoid foramen medially and covers the facial nerve exit. Before the age of 2 years, a retroauricular incision should not be extended inferiorly; otherwise the facial nerve could be injured at its exit from the stylomastoid foramen.

6.1.1   Facial Nerve Connections

At the 7th week, a ventral offshoot from the geniculate ganglion reaches the glossopharyngeal ganglion. This will form the lesser superficial petrosal nerve. At approximately the same time, the branch of the stapedial muscle appears [4].

Between the 12th and 13th week, two twigs from the dorsomedial surface of the facial nerve between the stapedial muscle and the chorda tympani nerve fuse together and reach the superior ganglia of the vagus (CN X) and glossopharyngeal (CN IX) nerves to give Arnold's nerve or the auricular branch of the vagus nerve. The Arnold's nerve traverses the primitive tympanomastoid

fissure and innervates the subcutaneous tissue of the posterior aspect of the external auditory canal (Ramsay Hunt area) [4].

By the 17th week, the definitive communications of the facial nerve, including those with the second and third cervical nerves, the trigeminal nerve, the vagus nerve, and the glossopharyngeal nerve, are established.

Clinical Applications
Facial Nerve in Aural Atresia

Facial nerve abnormal trajectory is common in major aural ear atresia. This is due to the abnormal development of the tympanic bone, which normally pushes the mastoid segment of the facial nerve posteriorly. The facial nerve may be placed in the middle ear cavity, mostly between the oval and the round windows (Fig. 6.5) [5].

6.2   Facial Nerve Anatomy

The facial nerve is the nerve of the second branchial arch. It contains motor and somatosensory components. The somatosensory component of the facial nerve is described under the name of the nervus intermedius, pars intermedia of Wrisberg.

The facial nerve is composed of approximately 10,000 neurons:

- 7,000 myelinated neurons: to form the motor part of the facial nerve that innervates the expressions muscles of the face and the stapedial muscle.
- 3,000 neurons: to form the nervus intermedius with secretory and somatosensory components. They include:
  1. The afferent taste fibers from the *chorda tympani* nerve, coming from the anterior two-thirds of the tongue
  2. The afferent taste fibers from the soft palate via the *palatine* and *greater petrosal* nerves
  3. The *parasympathetic secretory* innervations to the submandibular, sublingual, and lacrimal glands

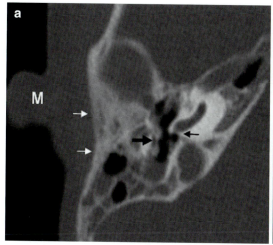 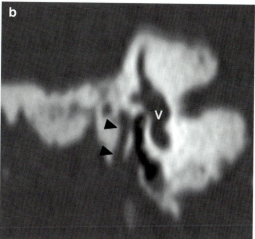

Fig. 6.5 (**a**) A transversal computed tomographic view of a right ear microtia and complete absence of the external auditory canal, atretic bony plate (*white arrows*). The mastoid segment of the facial nerve (*thick black arrow*) is displaced anteriorly, facing the round window (*thin black arrow*). *M* microtia. (**b**) Coronal view of an atretic ear showing the mastoid segment of the facial nerve (*arrowheads*) displaced anteriorly at the level of the vestibule (*V*)

4. The *cutaneous sensory* component from afferent fibers originating from the skin of the auricle and postauricular area or Ramsay Hunt area [6]

The facial nerve exits the brainstem at the pontomedullary junction; it traverses the cerebellopontine angle (CPA) and enters the internal auditory canal (IAC). Then it traverses the temporal bone in a bony canal, the Fallopian canal, until it reaches the stylomastoid foramen where it exits the temporal bone and enters the parotid gland [7, 8].

6.2.1 The Cerebellopontine Angle (CPA) Segment

The facial nerve (CN VII) leaves the brainstem at the pontomedullary junction almost 1.5 mm anterior to the vestibulocochlear nerve (VIII) [9].

The facial nerve then follows a rostro-lateral course through the cerebellopontine cistern for a distance of 15–17 mm, to enter finally the porus of the internal auditory canal (IAC) in the temporal bone.

The CPA segment of the facial nerve is 1.8 mm in diameter and is smaller than the cochleovestibular nerve CN VIII which is of around 3 mm [9]. A third smaller nerve, the nervus intermedius, emerges between CN VII and CN VIII.

> **Clinical Application**
> The root exit zone of the facial nerve (REZ) corresponds to a junctional area between central and peripheral myelin. At this level the facial nerve is sensitive to compression from a vascular loop; vascular compression at the REZ of the facial nerve is the most acceptable underlying physiopathology of a hemifacial spasm [10–13].

6.2.2 The Internal Auditory Canal Segment (IAC)

The IAC segment of the facial nerve occupies the anterosuperior quadrant of the IAC and measures 8–10 mm; it lies superior to the cochlear nerve and it passes above the crista falciformis [14]. The nervus intermedius passes between the motor root of the facial nerve and the cochlear nerve.

A crest of bone, the "Bill's bar" hangs in the vertical plane of the IAC between the superior vestibular nerve and the facial nerve, the later being anterior to the vestibular nerve (Fig. 6.6).

At the bottom of the IAC, the fundus, the facial nerve enters the Fallopian canal. This transit zone between the IAC and the Fallopian canal

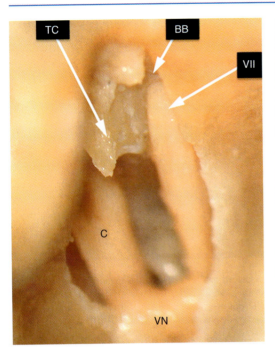

Fig. 6.6 Left ear translabyrinthine approach to the internal auditory canal after cut and reflection of both vestibular nerves (*VN*), showing the facial nerve (*VII*) lying superiorly and the cochlear nerve (*C*) inferiorly (the VII is anterior to the vestibular nerve). Bills bar (*BB*) is present in the meatus of the internal auditory canal and seperates the facial nerve from the superior vestibular nerve. *TC* tansverse crest (Courtesy of Tardivet [45])

is called the meatal segment and is the narrowest zone of bony facial canal; it is around 0.65 mm in diameter [14]. At this zone, the sheath of the nerve is formed only of pia mater and an arachnoid membrane because the dural investment terminates at the fundus of the IAC. This segment of the facial nerve is the most common site of entrapment during inflammatory disorders of the facial nerve, such as Bell's palsy and Ramsay Hunt syndrome.

6.2.3 The Facial Canal (Fallopian Aqueduct)

The facial nerve enters in a bony canal called the Fallopian canal (after Gabriel Fallopius). It is 25–30 mm in length [7]. No other nerve in the body travels such a long distance through a bony canal.

The Fallopian canal is divided into three distinct anatomic segments separated by two genus:

6.2.3.1 The Labyrinthine Segment (First Segment)

The labyrinthine segment of the facial nerve is 3–5 mm long; it is the shortest and the narrowest segment of the Fallopian canal. The narrowest part is at its entrance, the meatal segment. It lies beneath the middle cranial fossa and extends from the meatal foramen to the geniculate ganglion [15]. It travels anteriorly, superiorly, and laterally, forming an anteromedial angle of 120° with the IAC portion. It lies immediately above the anterior part of the vestibule.

The basal turn of the cochlea is anteroinferior to the labyrinthine segment and is in close relationship to the Fallopian canal.

When the nerve reaches a point just lateral and superior to the cochlea, it angles sharply forward, nearly at a right angles to the long axis of the petrous bone, to reach the geniculate ganglion (Fig. 6.7).

Before reaching the geniculate ganglion, both the facial nerve and the nervus intermedius remain distinct entities, and they meet each other just before joining the geniculate ganglion.

6.2.3.2 Geniculate Ganglion

The geniculate ganglion is situated at the lateral end of the labyrinthine segment. The pain fibers of the auricular branch and the taste fibers of the

Fig. 6.7 Middle cranial fossa view of a right-side facial nerve after drilling the bone covering the labyrinth, the facial nerve, and the tegmen tympani. *IAC* internal auditory canal segment of the facial nerve, *1* labyrinthine segment, *G* geniculate ganglion, *GSPN* greater superficial petrosal nerve, *2* tympanic segment, *Co* cochlear area, *M* malleus, *I* incus, * cochleariform process *LSCC* lateral semicircular canal, *PSCC* posterior semicircular cana, *SSCC* superior semicircular canall. (Courtesy of Tardivet [45])

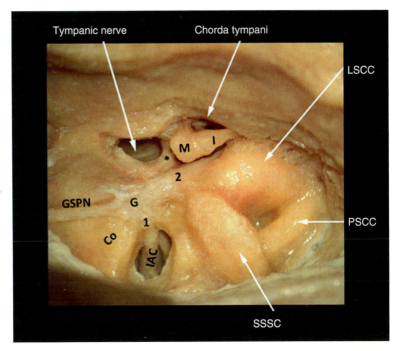

chorda tympani synapse with the second sensory neuron at the level of the geniculate ganglion; the secretomotor fibers to the lacrimal gland pass through the geniculate ganglion and form the greater petrosal superficial nerve.

At the level of the geniculate ganglion, the facial nerve takes an abrupt posterior direction, forming an acute angle 48–86° between the first and the second segment of the facial nerve; this is the "first genu" of the facial nerve [16] (Figs. 6.7 and 6.8). The geniculate ganglion is dehiscent in 15 % of temporal bones, a condition which makes the facial nerve vulnerable to injury during middle cranial fossa surgery.

6.2.3.3 The Greater Superficial Petrosal Nerve

The greater superficial petrosal nerve (GPSN) is a secretomotor branch of the facial nerve. It emerges from the anterior upper portion of the ganglion; it carries secretory fibers to the lacrimal glands. This nerve exits the petrous temporal bone in an anterointernal direction through the *hiatus of the facial canal* to enter the middle cranial fossa (Figs. 6.7 and 6.11).

In the middle cranial fossa, the GSPN passes deep to the Gasserian ganglion to reach the foramen lacerum where it enters the pterygoid canal. In the pterygoid canal, the GSPN joins the deep petrosal nerve to become the nerve of the pterygoid canal or vidian nerve. This nerve traverses the pterygoid canal and then the sphenopalatine ganglion, where the sensory fibers have their cell bodies. These fibers are distributed to the soft palate and to the tongue. Preganglionic secretory fibers from the cell bodies in the superior salivary nucleus also end in the sphenopalatine ganglion. Their corresponding postganglionic fibers innervate the lacrimal gland and provide secretory innervations to the nasal cavity.

The greater superficial petrosal canal also contains the superficial petrosal artery that supplies the geniculate ganglion region (see Sect. 6.2.3.8).

6.2.3.4 The Tympanic Segment (Second Segment)

The tympanic segment of the facial nerve extends from the geniculate ganglion anteriorly to the second genu of the facial nerve posteriorly. The tympanic segment inclines inferiorly and posteriorly to descend obliquely along the medial wall of the tympanic cavity, above the cochleariform process and the oval window and below the bulge

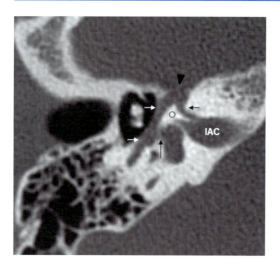

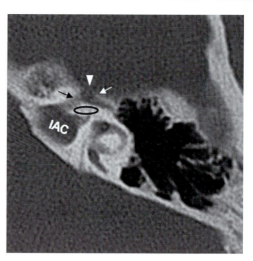

Fig. 6.8 Transversal computed tomographic view on a left ear. Labyrinthine segment (*short black arrow*), geniculate ganglion (*black arrowhead*), tympanic segment of the facial nerve (*white arrows*), oval window niche (*long black arrow*). Notice the acute angle between the first and second segment of the facial nerve (*circle*). *IAC* internal auditory canal

Fig. 6.9 Transversal computed tomography of a left ear showing a widened angle (*oval*) between the labyrinthine (*black arrow*) and tympanic segment (*white arrow*) of the facial nerve, suggesting a Gusher syndrome. Geniculate ganglion (*white arrowhead*). Note the bulbous aspect of the IAC

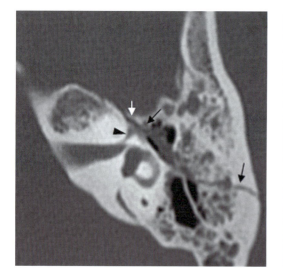

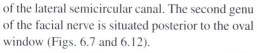

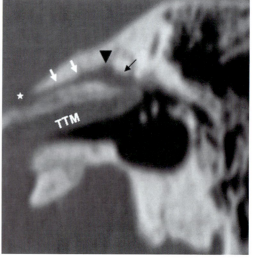

Fig. 6.10 Transversal computed tomographic view of a left ear with a longitudinal temporal bone fracture (*black arrows*), transgressing the geniculate ganglion (*white arrow*). Labyrinthine segment of the facial nerve (*arrowhead*)

Fig. 6.11 Sagittal reconstruction of a computed tomography. Facial nerve (*black arrow*), leaving the geniculate ganglion (*black arrowhead*) posteriorly. Greater superior petrosal nerve (*white arrows*) leaving the geniculate ganglion anteriorly. Hiatus of the facial canal (*), TTM tensor tympani muscle

of the lateral semicircular canal. The second genu of the facial nerve is situated posterior to the oval window (Figs. 6.7 and 6.12).

The length of the tympanic segment of the facial nerve varies between 9 and 12 mm. The width of the tympanic segment varies between 1.2 and 1.6 mm [16].

The anterior part of the tympanic segment of the facial nerve lies slightly above and medial to

In Gusher syndrome, an X-linked congenital mixed deafness, the IAC is abnormally wide. This creates a communication between the high-pressure cerebrospinal fluid in the IAC and the perilymph of the inner ear, leading to a leakage, the "stapes gusher," during stapes surgery. The pathological widening concerns also the Fallopian canal. The enlarged IAC may be seen on CT scan, with a globulous aspect, but this aspect is not specific. The widened angle between the first and the second segment of the facial nerve is highly suggestive of the Gusher syndrome, enabling the preoperative diagnosis of this pathology [17, 18] (Fig. 6.9).

The perigeniculate area is the weakest zone of the Fallopian canal; it is the most common localization of traumatic facial nerve injury in temporal bone fracture [19] (Fig. 6.10). It is of interest to note that compression of the nerve due to the bony spicules occurs much more frequently than nerve transaction.

- The greater superficial petrosal nerve represents an important landmark for facial nerve identification during middle cranial fossa approach.
- The section of the greater petrosal nerve or the section of vidian nerve has been proposed in the past to treat intractable vasomotor rhinitis; this surgery was abandoned because of its troublesome side effects of such reduction of the lacrimal secretions (dry eyes).

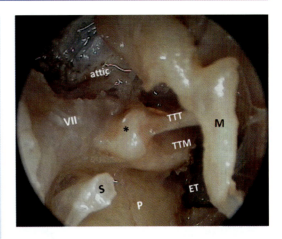

Fig. 6.12 Endoscopic view of a right middle ear through a posterior tympanotomy showing the tympanic segment of the facial nerve (*VII*) and its relationship with the cochleariform process (*) and stapes and oval window (*S*). *TTM* tensor tympani muscle, *TTT* tensor tympani tendon, *P* promontory, *ET* Eustachian tube, *M* malleus

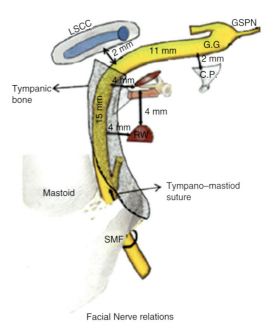

Fig. 6.13 Tympanomastoid segments of the facial nerve and their relationship to the middle ear structures. *GSPN* greater superficial petrosal nerve, *GG* geniculate ganglia, *CP* cochleariform process, *RW* round window, *LSCC* lateral semicircular canal, *SMF* stylomastoid foramen

the cochleariform process [13]. The relationship between the facial nerve and the cochleariform process is stable and constant. The cochleariform process is resistant to necrosis even in the presence of aggressive otitis media or cholesteatoma; therefore, it remains a persistent landmark helping to localize the facial nerve. The mean distance between the tympanic segment and the cochleariform process is around 2 mm (Fig. 6.13).

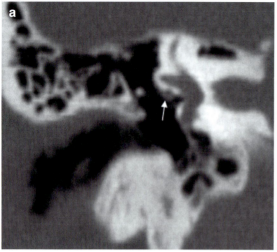 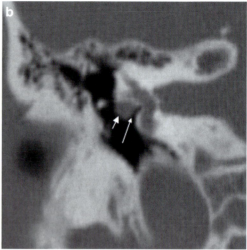

Fig. 6.14 Transversal computed tomographic views of the right ear showing (**a**) moderate prolapse of the tympanic segment of the facial nerve (*arrow*). (**b**) A bulging tympanic segment of the facial nerve (*short arrow*), obstructing almost completely the oval window niche (*long arrow*)

The mean distance between the second genu of the facial nerve and the oval window is of 3–4 mm [16] (Fig. 6.13). The tympanic segment of the facial nerve courses posteriorly below and medial to the bulging of the lateral semicircular canal and not far from the pyramidal process [19, 20].

The bony wall of the tympanic segment canal can be very thin or even dehiscent, and the middle ear mucosa may lay in direct contact with the facial nerve sheath [21, 22].

Within the Fallopian canal, bundles of nerve fibers lie in a definite order. The oral branche lies next to the oval window, the frontal branches farthest from it, and the ocular branches in between [23, 24].

The lateral bony wall of the nerve is well visualized by CT scan. Dehiscence of the inferior wall may be difficult to assess correctly on the coronal views, but these views are demonstrative for the different degrees of prolapse of the facial nerve in front of the oval window niche or even in close contact to the stapes (Fig. 6.14).

6.2.3.5 Second Genu

The second genu is the junction between the tympanic and the mastoid segments of the facial nerve. Just lateral and posterior to the pyramidal eminence, the facial nerve changes its direction and courses inferiorly about 2–3 mm to form an angulation of about 90–125° called the second genu. The second genu lies inferior to the lateral semicircular canal and medial to the short process of the incus. The mean distance between the short process of the incus and the second genu is a relatively constant relationship and it measures about 2 mm (Figs. 6.15 and 6.16).

Surgical Impacts

The second genu of the facial nerve is the most susceptible portion of the nerve to suffer from an iatrogenic injury during ear surgery because it is not visible before identifying the nerve itself, especially in cases of invasive cholesteatoma and granulation tissue.

Knowing that the second genu is located inferior and medial to the aditus, the nerve could be at risk of injury while drilling towards the aditus during mastoid surgery. A sclerotic mastoid or the presence of extended chronic ear pathologies may hinder the proper identification of the anatomical structures bordering the aditus and expose the facial nerve to a risk of injury [19].

Fig. 6.15 Transmastoid view of a left ear after posterior and anterior tympanotomy, showing the relationship between the lateral semicircular canal (*) and the second genu of the facial nerve between the tympanic segment (*2*) and the mastoid segments (*3*) of facial nerve. *GG* geniculate ganglia, *1* labyrinthine segment of the facial nerve, *SPI* short process of the incus (Courtesy of Tardivet [45])

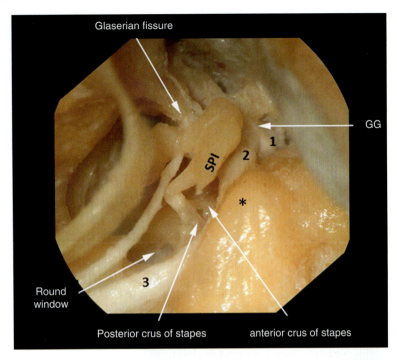

Glaserian fissure

GG

SPI

2

1

*

Round window

3

Posterior crus of stapes

anterior crus of stapes

6.2.3.6 The Mastoid Segment (Third Segment)

The mastoid segment of the facial nerve is the longest part of the intra-temporal part of the facial nerve. This segment is vertical and lengths about 15 mm [20]. The mastoid Fallopian canal is relatively the largest part of the Fallopian canal; the nerve fills only 25–50 % of the Fallopian canal lumen at this level. Inflammatory entrapment of the facial nerve is rare in the mastoid segment [25, 26].

The mastoid segment descends downwards in the posterior wall of the tympanic cavity from the second genu superiorly to the stylomastoid foramen inferiorly. As the nerve descends inferiorly towards the mastoid tip, it becomes more lateral. In many cases, the inferior portion of the mastoid segment may course lateral to the plane of the postero-inferior quadrant of the annulus [27] (Fig. 6.17).

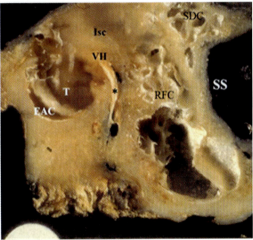

SDC

lsc

VII

T

*

RFC

SS

EAC

Fig. 6.16 A sagittal cut of a left middle ear in the plane of mastoid segment of facial nerve (*); notice the relationship between the second genu (*VII*) and the lateral semicircular canal (*lsc*); retrofacial cells (*RFC*) separate the sigmoid sinus (*SS*) from the facial nerve. *SDC* sino-dural angle cells, *T* tympanic cavity, *EAC* external auditory canal

> **Clinical Impact**
> During canaloplasty, the annulus should not be considered as a secure landmark for facial nerve; the facial nerve may pass lateral to the annulus [27]. In such cases, drilling in the posteroinferior quadrant of the external auditory canal, even lateral to the annulus, may lead to a facial nerve injury.

Relationship Between the Mastoid Segment of the Facial Nerve and the Tympanum

The mastoid segment of the facial nerve lies in the posterior wall of the tympanum in a position lateral to the pyramidal process, stapedial muscle, and the sinus tympani. The mean distance between the mastoid segment of the facial nerve and the posterior border of the oval window is

Fig. 6.17 Right ear after dissection of the mastoid segment of the facial nerve (*VII*), showing its relation with tympanic annulus (*); notice that the inferior portion of the mastoid facial nerve is lateral to annulus. *CT* chorda tympani, *LSCC* lateral semicircular canal, *PSCC* posterior semicircular canal, *I* incus short process

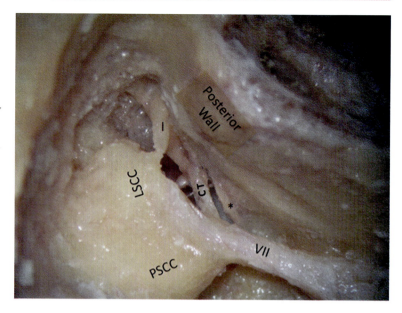

4 mm. Also the distance between the facial nerve and the round window is 4 mm (Fig. 6.13). In addition, the minimal distance from the annulus tympanicus to the facial nerve is about 1 mm at 9 o'clock position [16]. This fact permits to increase surgically the dimensions of the posterior tympanotomy by sacrificing the chorda tympani nerve (see Chap. 4).

Relationship Between the Mastoid Segment of the Facial Nerve and the Mastoid Structures
In the mastoid cavity, the mastoid segment runs straight downwards from below the most overlapping part of the lateral semicircular canal to the stylomastoid foramen. The nerve is surrounded by the compacta of the bony wall of the ear canal and by mastoid sells. Occasionally, there is a bony defect in the Fallopian canal and the nerve is dehiscent into the mastoid air cells.

The lower one-third of the mastoid segment of the facial nerve is always medial and anterior to the digastric ridge which represents an important landmark for the facial nerve exposure in a lateral skull base approaches (Fig. 6.18). Nevertheless the digastric ridge may be difficult to identify when the mastoid is poorly pneumatized.

The sigmoid sinus passes always posterior and medial to the facial nerve. The distance between the mastoid segment and the sigmoid sinus is highly variable (4 mm average). The distance from the facial nerve to the jugular bulb ranges from 0 to 12 mm [16].

The facial nerve exits the Fallopian canal via the stylomastoid foramen. The mean depth of the facial nerve from the mastoid cortex at the stylomastoid foramen is 13 mm. As the nerve exits the stylomastoid foramen at the anterior margin of the digastric groove, an adherent fibrous sheath of dense vascularized connective tissue surrounds it. The stylomastoid artery and veins are within this dense sheath. When it exits the stylomastoid foramen, the nerve travels between the digastric and stylohyoid muscles and enters the parotid gland.

Below the stylomastoid foramen, a sensory branch emerges from the facial nerve to innervate the posterior wall of the external auditory canal and a portion of the tympanic membrane.

The superior landmarks for the mastoid segment of the facial nerve are the lateral semicircular canal, to which the facial nerve runs anteroinferiorly, and the posterior semicircular canal, to which the nerve runs 2.5 mm anteriorly. The digastric ridge is the inferior landmark

Fig. 6.18 Cadaveric left mastoidectomy showing the mastoid segment of the facial nerve (*VII*). Notice that the VII is anteromedial to the digastric ridge (*D*). The relationship between the tympanic annulus (*a*), chorda tympani (*CT*), and VII. The second genu of the facial nerve passes medial to the short process of the incus (*I*) and the lateral semicircular canal (*LSSC*); the VII drops down in the mastoid at the level of the midpoint of the LSCC in a direction parallel to that of the short process of the incus. * incudal buttress

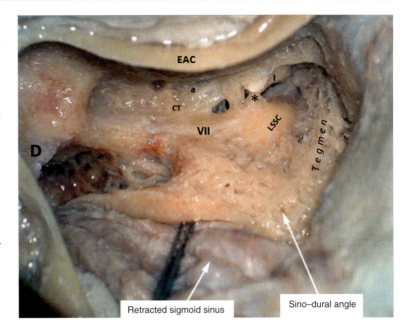

6.2.3.7 Mastoid Segment Branches

Two branches exit the mastoid segment of the facial nerve: the stapedial muscle nerve and the chorda tympani nerve.

The Nerve of Stapedial Muscle

The nerve fibers of the stapedial muscle arise centrally from some neurons emerging outside the nucleus of the facial nerve and are situated below the IV ventricle to join secondarily the motor neurons of the facial nerves [29, 30].

The nerve of the stapedial muscle is a small twig coming from the facial nerve as it descends in the posterior wall of the tympanic cavity behind the pyramidal eminence.

> *Clinical Notes*
> The distinct central origin of the stapedial nerve explains the normal finding of stapedial muscle reflex in congenital facial palsy (Mobius syndrome) and the isolated alteration of stapedial reflex without facial palsy in some brain stem lesions.

The Chorda Tympani

The chorda tympani is the terminal branch of the nervus intermedius. The chorda tympani

for the mastoid segment of the facial nerve. It is a smooth convex bone found close to the mastoid tip.

> *Surgical Applications*
> **Mastoid Segment Identification During Mastoid Surgery**
> Exposure of the facial nerve is done through a cortical mastoidectomy. The most important landmarks for identifying the facial nerve in the mastoid cavity are the horizontal semicircular canal, the short process of the incus, and the digastric ridge [28]. The axis of the VII corresponds to the axis of the short process of the incus.
>
> The nerve is best identified by first imagining a line that begins just anterior to the inferior portion of the lateral semicircular canal and travels in an inferior direction towards the digastric ridge. The bone of the EAC is progressively thinned, in a direction parallel to the nerve, until the white sheath is identified through the yellow bone.
>
> The drilling must be always done along the lateral aspect of the nerve, not behind and medial to the Fallopian canal.

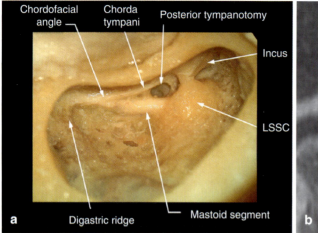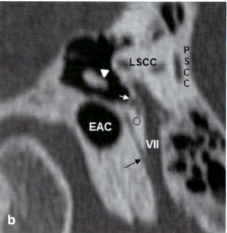

Fig. 6.19 (**a**) Left ear: cadaveric cut of a left ear showing the chordo-facial angle of Plester (Courtesy of Tardivet [45]). (**b**) Sagittal reconstruction of a computed tomography showing the emergence of the chorda (*black arrow*) from the facial nerve (*VII*) and the bony wall (*circle*) between the chorda and the VII (facial recess approach). Facial recess (*white arrow*), short process of the incus (*white arrowhead*), *LSCC* lateral semicircular canal, *PSCC* posterior semicircular canal, *EAC* external auditory canal

leaves the mastoid segment of the facial nerve at a variable level, about 5–6 mm above the stylomastoid foramen. The facial nerve and the chorda tympani emergence form the Plester's chordo-facial angle which varies between 26° and 35° (Fig. 6.19) [16].

The chorda tympani enters the middle ear through the chordal eminence. It passes between the incus and the handle of the malleus, above the tensor tympani tendon to exit through the canal of Huguier of the petrotympanic fissure. Then the chorda tympani passes on the medial surface of the mandibular fossa to finally join the lingual nerve in the infratemporal fossa (Fig. 6.20) [31].

The chorda tympani nerve carries:

- *Sensory afferent taste fibers*: these fibers of the chorda tympani nerve have their cell bodies in the geniculate ganglion and provide taste sensation from the anterior two-thirds of the tongue.
- *Preganglionic efferent secretory fibers* to the submaxillary and sublingual glands: these fibers have their cell bodies in the superior salivary nucleus; they synapse within the submaxillary ganglion, and then it provides secretory motor impulses to the submaxillary and sublingual glands.

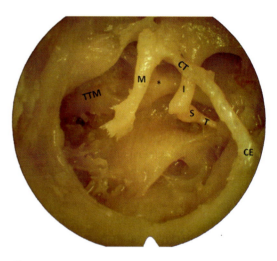

Fig. 6.20 Endoscopic view of a left middle ear showing the chorda tympani (*CT*) entering the middle ear through the chordal eminence (*C.E.*); it then passes between incus (*I*) medially and the malleus (*M*) laterally, above the tensor tympani tendon (***) to exit the middle ear from the anterior wall. *T* stapedial tendon, *S* stapes, *TTM* tensor tympani muscle

---

Surgical Impact

Chorda Tympani Nerve (CT) Injury During Middle Ear Surgery

Iatrogenic chorda tympani nerve (CTN) injury during middle ear surgery is quite

Fig. 6.21 Tympanomastoid segment vascularization. *1* stylomastoid artery, *2* superficial petrosal artery *LSCC* lateral semicircular canal; *OW* oval window; *RW* round window; *TTM* tensor tympani muscle; *STR* supratubal recess; *AE* anterior epitympanum; *GG* geniculate ganglion; *GSPN* greater superficial petrosal nerve

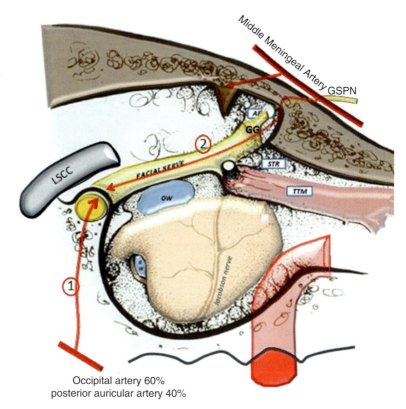

Occipital artery 60%
posterior auricular artery 40%

common. The most frequent type of chorda tympani injury is stretching, cutting the nerve is less common. Canal wall down mastoidectomy and posterior tympanotomy have the highest risk of chorda tympani injury [32].

Only 25 % of patients are aware of the symptoms after chorda tympani injury. Stretching or cutting the chorda tympani could give the same types of symptoms to the concerned patients.

Additional studies demonstrated that nerve stretching is associated with a greater degree of postoperative symptoms than nerve transsection, across a range of middle ear procedures [32, 33].

Nevertheless, these finding are in contrast to the results of testing the taste disturbance after stapedectomy, in which cutting of the nerve was found to cause significantly greater symptoms than manipulation alone [34].

The most common postoperative complaint is taste disturbance such a metallic taste. Although most patients experience gradual symptomatic recovery, about 90 % of the symptomatic patients recover completely within 12 months. Persisting complaints may be troublesome [35]. The risk of taste disturbance should be addressed in the consent procedure.

6.2.4 Vascularization of the Facial Nerve (Fig. 6.21)

The segments of the facial nerve receive their arterial supply from branches of the vertebrobasilar artery and the external carotid artery systems. Within the pons, the facial nucleus receives its blood supply primarily from the anterior inferior cerebellar artery (AICA). The labyrinthine artery, a branch of the AICA, enters the internal auditory canal (IAC) with the facial nerve and provides blood supply to the meatal portion of the facial nerve.

The external carotid system gives to the tympanomastoid segments of the facial nerve two branches: the superficial petrosal artery and the stylomastoid artery.

6.2.4.1 Superficial Petrosal Artery

The superficial petrosal artery is an endocranial branch of the middle meningeal artery (MMA); it enters the middle ear through the facial hiatus with the greater superficial petrosal nerve. It supplies the geniculate ganglion and the tympanic segment of the facial nerve. It anastomoses with the stylomastoid artery at the level of the second genu.

6.2.4.2 Stylomastoid Artery

The stylomastoid artery arises from the external carotid artery system; it enters the middle ear and the facial canal through the stylomastoid foramen. It supplies the mastoid segment of the facial nerve. It anastomoses with the superficial petrosal artery of the MMA at the level of the second genu [36].

In 60 % of patients, the stylomastoid artery arises from the occipital artery and in 40 % of patients it arises from the postauricular artery [37].

The superficial petrosal artery and the stylomastoid artery contribute to an arterial arcade called the facial arch which supplies the tympanic and mastoid segments of the facial nerve. In most people this arcade is supplied predominantly by the superficial petrosal artery [38] (Fig. 6.21).

Furthermore, 10 % of people lack a blood supply from the MMA to the geniculate ganglion, meaning that the mastoid and tympanic segments receive their blood supply only from the stylomastoid artery [39].

Clinical Implications

In lateral skull base surgery, anterior and posterior rerouting of the facial nerve reduces drastically the blood supply of the facial nerve with a high risk of facial weakness. The blood supply of the mastoid segment of the facial nerve maintains adherent this portion to the canal, a point to take in consideration when dissecting the nerve from the canal [40].

Embolization in the territories of the external carotid artery is commonly indicated to treat vascular lesions including intractable epistaxis, hypervascular neoplasms, dural fistulae, and arteriovenous malformations.

When a dual blood supply of the tympanomastoid segments of the facial nerve is present, a supraselective embolization (SSE), with occlusion of the stylomastoid artery, would not be at risk to induce paresis. However, in cases of an absent blood supply derivative from the MMA, embolization of the stylomastoid artery would likely result in a facial nerve deficit.

Since 6 % of patients would be expected to derive their blood supply of the facial nerve tympanomastoid segments only from the stylomastoid artery originating from the occipital artery, patients undergoing supraselective embolization of the stylomastoid artery should be counseled on a theoretical 6 % risk of having a vascular anatomic pattern that may place the facial nerve at increased risk during embolization [41].

The embolization agent, such as nonabsorbable polymers, also influences the risk of developing a cranial neuropathy [42].

Considering this risk, catheterizing the MMA is suggested to assess the length of the superficial petrosal artery [42]. If a dual blood supply to the facial nerve is confirmed, there is no risk of facial nerve paresis from embolization. But if the superficial petrosal artery branch is short, resorbable agents should be considered.

Symptoms from ischemic facial nerve palsy during embolization of the external carotid artery branches occur immediately following the procedure and may be not fully recoverable [43]. Facial nerve decompression is one of several strategies for restoring nerve function in case of acute nerve palsy [44].

References

1. Louryan S. Développement du nerf facial. In: Martin-Duverneuil N, editor. A propos du nerf facial. Paris: Guerbet; 1994. p. 3–9.
2. Bast TH, Anson BJ, Richany SF. The development of the second branchial arch (Reichert's cartilage), facial canal and associated structures in man. Q Bull Northwest Univ Med Sch. 1956;30:235–49.
3. Spector JG, Ge X. Ossification patterns of the tympanic facial canal in the human fetus and neonate. Laryngoscope. 1993;103:1052–65.
4. GulyaIn AJ. Developmental anatomy of the temporal bone and skull base. In: Glasscock-Shambaugh's surgery of the ear. 6th ed. Shelton: People's Medical Publishing House; 2010. p. 3–27.
5. Wetmore RF, Muntz HR, McGill TJ. Pediatric otolaryngology: principles and practice pathways. New York: Thieme Medical Publishers; 2000.
6. http://emedicine.medscape.com/article/835286-overview
7. Chandra S, Goyal M, Gandhi D, Gera S, Berry M. Anatomy of the facial nerve in the temporal bone: HRCT. Indian J Radiol Imaging. 1999;9(1):5–8.
8. Cornelia U, editor. Paralizii le nervu lui facial. Laşi: Ars Longa; 2001. p. 11–7.
9. Gantz Bruce J, Rubinstein Jay T. Intratemporal facial nerve surgery. In: CW Cummings, JM Fredrickson, LA Harker, CJ Krause, MA Richardson, DE Schuller, editors. Otolaryngology head and neck surgery. 3rd ed. St. Louis: Mosby—Year Book, Inc.; 1998. Vol 4(143). p. 2785–99.
10. Magnan J, Chays A. [Functional surgery on the acoustic-facial pedicle]. Rev Laryngol Otol Rhinol (Bord). 1998;119(3):151–4. Review. French.
11. Magnan J, Caces F, Locatelli P, Chays A. Hemifacial spasm: endoscopic vascular decompression. Otolaryngol Head Neck Surg. 1997;117(4):308–14.
12. Badr-El-Dine M, El-Garem HF, Talaat AM, Magnan J. Endoscopically assisted minimally invasive microvascular decompression of hemifacial spasm. Otol Neurotol. 2002;23(2):122–8.
13. Magnan J, Chays A, Caces F, Lepetre-Gillot C, Cohen JM, Belus JF, et al. Role of endoscopy and vascular decompression in the treatment of hemifacial spasm. Ann Otolaryngol Chir Cervicofac. 1994;111(3):153–60. French.
14. Ge XX, Spector GJ. Labyrinthine segment and geniculate ganglion of the facial nerve in fetal and adult temporal bones. Ann Otol Rhinol Laryngol. 1981;90 suppl 85:1–12.
15. Proctor B. Surgical anatomy of the ear and temporal bone. New York: Thieme Medical Publishers; 1989.
16. Măru N, Cheiţă AC, Mogoantă CA, Prejoianu B. Intratemporal course of the facial nerve: morphological, topographic and morphometric features. Rom J Morphol Embryol. 2010;51(2):243–8.
17. Kumar G, Castello M, Bucman CA. X-linked stapes gusher; CT findings in one patient. Am J Neuroradiol. 2003;24:1130–2.
18. Talbot JM, Wilson DF. Computed tomographic diagnosis of X-linked congenital mixed deafness, fixation of the stapedial footplate, and perilymphatic gusher. Am J Otol. 1994;15(2):177–82.
19. Ozgirgin N, Cenjor C, Filipo R, Magnan J. Consensus on treatment algorithms for traumatic and iatrogenic facial paralysis. Mediterr J Otol. 2007;3:150–8.
20. Yadav S, Ranga A, Sirohiwal B. Surgical anatomy of tympano-mastoid segment of facial nerve. Indian J Otolaryngol Head Neck Surg. 2006;58(1):27–30.
21. Baxter A. Dehiscence of the fallopian canal. An anatomical study. J Laryngol Otol. 1971;85(6):587–94.
22. Kim CW, Rho YS, Ahn HY, Oh SJ. Facial canal dehiscence in the initial operation for chronic otitis media without cholesteatoma. Auris Nasus Larynx. 2008;35(3):353–6.
23. Miehlke A. Uber die Topographie des Faserverlaufes im Facialisstamm. Arch Ohren Nasen Kehlkopfheilkd. 1958;171:340.
24. Hofmann L. Der Faserverlauf im N. facialis. Z Hals Nas Ohrenheilk. 1924;10:86.
25. Jongkees LBW. Die chirurgische Behandlung der intrtemporalen Facialishahmung. Dtsch Med Wochenschr. 1958;83:865.
26. Lindemann H. The fallopian canal. An anatomical study of its distal part. Acta Otolaryngol Suppl. 1960;158:204.
27. Adad B, Rasgon BM, Ackerson L. Relationship of the facial nerve to the tympanic annulus: a direct anatomic examination. Laryngoscope. 1999;109(8):1189–92.
28. Chi FL, Wang J, Yuan YS, Liu HJ, Gu J, Huang T, et al. Landmark of facial nerve in middle ear surgery. Zhonghua Er Bi Yan Hou Tou Jing Wai Ke Za Zhi. 2006;41(1):5–8.
29. Lyon MJ. The central location of the motor neurons to the stapedius muscle in the cat. Brain Res. 1978;143(3):437–44.
30. Joseph MP, Guinan Jr JJ, Fullerton BC, Norris BE, Kiang NY. Number and distribution of stapedius motoneurons in cats. J Comp Neurol. 1985;232:43–54.
31. Tóth M, Moser G, Patonay L, Oláh I. Development of the anterior chordal canal. Ann Anat. 2006;188(1):7–11.
32. Gopalan P, Kumar M, Gupta D, Phillips JJ. A study of chorda tympani nerve injury and related symptoms following middle-ear surgery. J Laryngol Otol. 2005;119(3):189–92.
33. Clark MP, O'Malley S. Chorda tympani nerve function at er middle ear surgery. Otol Neurotol. 2007;28(3):335–40.
34. Mahendran S, Hogg R, Robinson JM. To divide or manipulate the chorda tympani in stapedotomy. Eur Arch Otorhinolaryngol. 2005;262(6):482–7.
35. Kiverniti E, Watters G. Taste disturbance after mastoid surgery: immediate and long-term effects of chorda tympani nerve sacrifice. J Laryngol Otol. 2012;126(1):34–7.
36. Ozanne A, Pereira V, Krings T, et al. Arterial vascularization of the cranial nerves. Neuroimaging Clin N Am. 2008;18:431–9, xii.

37. Magnan J, Chays A, Gasquet R, Didier D, Garcia C, Bremond G. Anatomie chirurgicale de la tympanotomie postérieure. JF ORL. 1990;5:301–13.

38. Djindjian R, Merland JJ. Super-selective arteriography of the external carotid artery. Berlin: Springer; 1978. p. 14–123.

39. Marangos NM, Schumacher M. Facial palsy after glomus jugulare tumor embolization. J Laryngol Otol. 1999;113:268–70.

40. Sanna M, Khrais T, Mancini F, Russo A, Taibah A. The facial nerve in temporal bone and lateral skull base microsurgery. Stuttgart/New York: G Thieme Verlag; 2006.

41. Gartrell BC, Hansen MR, Gantz BJ, Gluth MB, Mowry SE, Aagaard-Kienitz BL, et al. Facial and lower cranial neuropathies after preoperative embolization of jugular foramen lesions with ethylene vinyl alcohol. Otol Neurotol. 2012;33(7):1270–5.

42. Valavanis A. Preoperative embolization of the head and neck: indications, patient selection, goals, and precautions. Am J Neuroradiol. 1986;7:943–52.

43. de Vries N, Versluis RJ, Valk J, et al. Facial nerve paralysis following embolization for severe epistaxis (case report and review of the literature). J Laryngol Otol. 1986;100:207–10.

44. Ramakrishnan Y, Alam S, Kotecha A, et al. Reanimation following facial palsy: present and future directions. J Laryngol Otol. 2010;124:1146–52.

45. Tardivet L. Anatomie Chirurgicale du nerf facial intrapetreux, Thèse Med. Aix Marseille University 2003.

The Eustachian Tube

7

Contents

The Eustachian tube (ET) or auditory tube is a slender tube that connects the middle ear cavity with the nasopharynx and serves to equalize air pressure on either side of the eardrum.

It is a hollow structure of bone and cartilage, lined with a mucous membrane, and equipped by a muscular opening mechanism.

It is part of a system of contiguous organs, including the nose, the middle ear, and the mastoid air cells. This system is devoted to middle ear ventilation, its protection, and its clearance. Impairment of this system leads to middle ear dysventilation, which is the primary cause of the development of chronic otitis media.

7.1 Eustachian Tube Development

The ET lumen develops from the persistence of the first pharyngeal pouch. Between the second and third week of gestation, the first pharyngeal pouch extends laterally between the first and the second branchial arches to make contact with the first branchial groove which is the origin of the external auditory meatus (Fig. 7.1). The distal part of this pouch expands to form the tubotympanic recess which is the primordium of the middle ear cavity. The proximal part becomes constricted to connect the future middle ear to the pharynx.

The structures associated with ET lumen develop from the mesenchyme surrounding the first pharyngeal pouch in a predictable sequence:

Fig. 7.1 The tubotympanic recess (TR) in a mouse embryo of gestation day 12. *HM* handle of malleus, *Ph* pharynx, *OC* otic capsule, *TTR* tubotympanic recess, *FBG* first branchial ectodermal groove. This horizontal section demonstrates the continuity between the pouch and the pharynx. Incorporation of radioactive sulfur with hematoxylin-eosin counterstaining

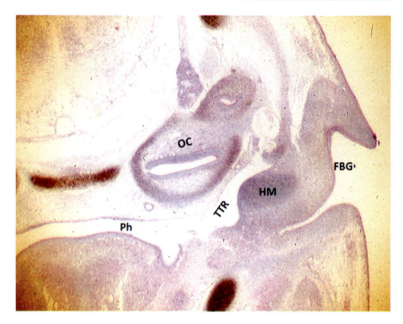

Fig. 7.2 Frontal section of the auditory tube rudiment in a 27-mm human embryo (end of the second month). *TVP* tensor veli palatine muscle anlage, *LVP* levator veli palatine muscle anlage. Hematoxylin-eosin staining

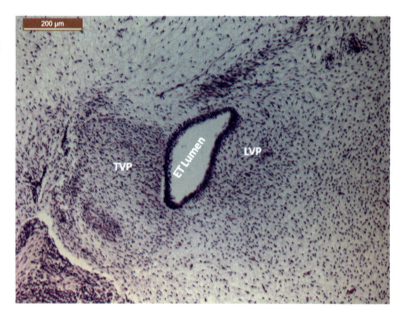

Before the 10th week of gestation, only the epithelial lining of the lumen has differentiated. Between the 10th and 12th week, the levator veli palatini (LVP) and tensor veli palatini muscles (TVP) develop and become delineated from the surrounding mesenchyme [1, 2] (Fig. 7.2).

The initial differentiation of the cartilage begins at the 14th week. By the 20th week, the initial center of chondrification has increased in size and a perichondrium is clearly differentiated in the anteromedial portion of the tube [1, 2] (Fig. 7.3).

These processes yield an ET structure very similar to that observed in an adult. Later during the rest of fetal life, morphometric changes occur among the ET structures. The most pronounced change is the increase in the length of the cartilaginous portion of the tube from 1 mm at the 10th week of gestation to 13 mm at birth.

Fig. 7.3 A transverse cut of the base of skull in a 6-month fetus showing the Eustachian tube. Note the cartilaginous part is well developed (*white arrows*) and is in the same plane as the bony Eustachian tube (*ET*). *LPM* lateral pterygoid muscle, *Sph* sphenoid bone, *ICA* internal carotid artery, *TVP* tensor veli palatini muscle

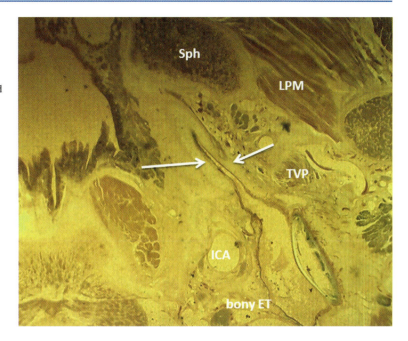

While the fetus is growing, the tube deviates from the horizontal plane only about 10°, because the fetal cranial base is relatively flat; this situation persists until early childhood [1–4].

> **Clinical Application**
> An arrest of the development of the tubotympanic recess when the normal constriction of the tube is deficient may lead to a persistent wide open Eustachian tube all over its length. This is illustrated in this case of an adult female of 35 years old (Fig. 7.4). The developmental arrest concerns the whole left ear, associated to microtia, and external auditory canal atresia.

7.1.1   Postnatal Growth (Fig. 7.5)

The ET lengthens rapidly during early childhood: In infants, it is about half as long as that in adults; it is about 18 mm [5] and it reaches adult size by 7 years of age [6, 7].

The cartilaginous portion increases dramatically: The ratio of the length of the cartilaginous portion to the osseous portion is 8:1 in the infant, but this ratio becomes 4:1 in the adult due to the growth of the bony portion [8].

In infants, the cartilaginous and bony portions are aligned with a line that connects the pharynx and middle ear; however, due to the craniofacial growth, the cartilaginous tube is angled inferiorly from the osseous portion to form an angle of approximately 45° related to the horizontal plane [1, 9].

The LVP muscle increases in cross-sectional area and in volume and assumes a more suitable vector for an efficient active tubal dilatation.

The ET of the infant is floppy, very distensible, and lacks recoil phenomena of the hinge region. With time, the tubal cartilage stiffens and the elastin component develops in the hinge region; this will result in a reduced tubal compliance and an increased recoil, which raise the protective mechanism of the ET [10].

The lumen of the ET increases almost five times from the newborn to persons aged 20 years old; the cross-sectional length of the lumen increases significantly with age, especially in the pharyngeal area of the tube.

The lumen in most of the cartilaginous portion of the ET is significantly smaller in children than in adults [11].

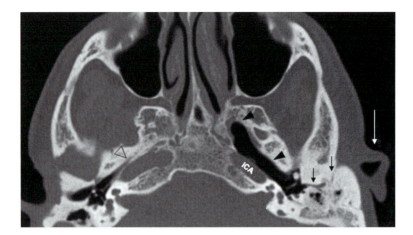

Fig. 7.4 Transversal computed tomographic view of both ears in a patient presenting left ear microtia (*white arrow*) and atresia of the external auditory canal (*black arrows*), also an abnormally large Eustachian tube (*arrow heads*) due to the arrest of constriction of the tubotympanic recess in contrast to the normal right side (*empty arrow head*). *ICA* internal carotid artery

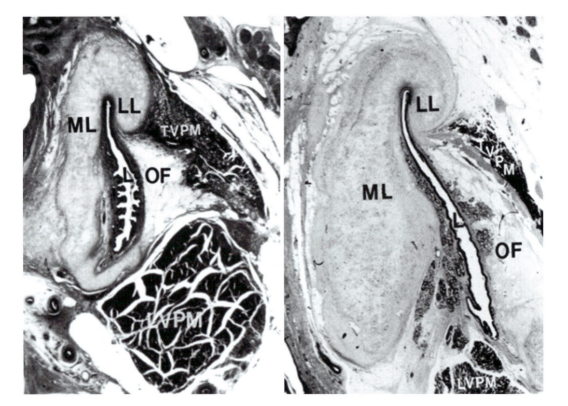

Fig. 7.5 Photomicrographs of cross sections through the midcartilaginous portion of the Eustachian tube (ET) of a 3-month-old female (*left*) and a 34-year-old male (*right*) showing the developmental difference of Ostmann's fat pad (*OF*) and the size of the ET. *L* lumen, *LL* lateral lamina of the Eustachian tube cartilage, *LVPM* levator veli palatini muscle, *ML* medial lamina of the Eustachian tube cartilage, *TVPM* tensor veli palatini muscle (Courtesy of I. Sando, MD) (Reproduced with permission from Eustachian tube: structure, Function, Role in otitis media, by Charles D. Bluestone. pmph-usa.com)

Also the Ostmann's fat pad increases in volume with age until adulthood, which may be related to better protective function in adults [12].

7.2   Eustachian Tube Anatomy

The ET is a narrow osteocartilaginous channel connecting the tympanic cavity to the nasopharynx. Its lumen allows the passage of two different physical substances: one is gaseous for middle ear ventilation, and the second is fluid for the middle ear clearance. The ET begins at the tympanic orifice of the protympanum and ends at the pharyngeal orifice situated on the lateral wall of the nasopharynx. During its trajectory, the tube takes a slow curving inverted S course.

The general shape of the ET resembles to an hourglass made of two unequal cones. The first is small and fix, the posterior third, and represents the bony ET. The other one is elongated and mobile, the anterior two-thirds, and represents the fibrocartilaginous ET. Both parts are connected at the junctional zone, forming an angle of 160°.

In adults, the tubal axis forms with the plane of the hard palate an average angle of 36°(range 31–40°); the total length of the ET is 33 mm, divided as the following: the cartilaginous part is of 23.5 mm, the junctional part is of 3 mm, and the bony part is of 6.5 mm [13, 14] (Fig. 7.6).

The bony portion is patent at all times; in contrary the fibrocartilaginous portion is closed at rest and opens intermittently.

7.2.1   The Bony Portion of the Eustachian Tube

The bony part of ET lies completely within the petrous part of the temporal bone. It runs from the tympanic orifice of the middle ear cavity in an anteromedial direction, following the petrous apex, towards the petrosphenoid sulcus on the inferior surface of the skull base.

The tympanic orifice of the Eustachian tube lies in the middle third of the anterior wall of the middle ear cavity, 4 mm above the floor of the middle ear and close to the carotid canal and the labyrinth (see Section 2.5.2). It is an oval

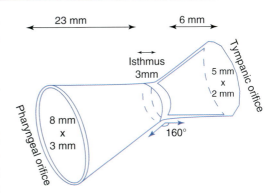

Fig. 7.6 Schematic drawing of different Eustachian tube dimensions (average)

structure that measures about 5 mm (horizontally) × 2 mm (vertically) [9] (Fig. 7.6).

Bony ET lumen is roughly triangular, measuring 2–3 mm vertically and 3–4 mm along the horizontal base [15].

The medial wall of the bony tube corresponds to the cochlea posteriorly and to the carotid canal anteriorly. The average thickness of the anteromedial portion of its bony wall is 1.5–3 mm. This bony wall is dehiscent in 2 % of individuals, exposing the carotid artery [15] (Fig. 7.7).

The upper third of the endoluminal surface of the medial wall presents the bony canal of the tensor tympani muscle. The lateral wall of the bony tube neighbors the canal of Hugier and the temporomandibular joint. The upper wall or roof of the bony tube corresponds to the tegmen tubari (Figs. 7.7 and 7.8).

On the inferior surface of the base of skull, the end of the bony tube is constricted and it opens on the posterior part of the tubal sulcus; the bony tube end is situated between the carotid canal medially and the temporomandibular joint laterally.

Surgical Implication
The majority of temporal bone with pneumatized petrous apex harbor peritubal air cells that may open directly into the ET lumen (Fig. 7.9). This explains the probability of cerebrospinal fluid rhinorrhea after translabyrinthine approach to the cerebellopontine angle when ET obliteration is not performed sufficiently far into the lumen by the end of the procedure [16].

Fig. 7.7 Transverse cut of a left ear showing the bony Eustachian tube (*Pr*) housing the tensor tympani muscle (*), the cartilaginous Eustachian tube (*ET*), and the isthmus (*I*). Notice the relation of the Eustachian tube and the cochlea (*C*) and the petrous internal carotid artery (*IC*) medially and the temporomandibular joint (*TMJ*) and middle meningeal artery (*ma*) laterally. *EAC* external auditory canal, *1* attic outer wall, *2* anterior wall of EAC, *3* posterior wall of the EAC, *m* malleus, *VII* tympanic segment of facial nerve, *CSCS* superior semicircular canal

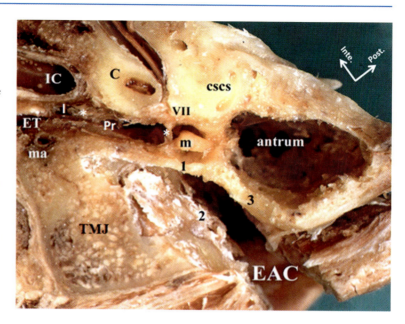

Fig. 7.8 Medial view of a sagittal cadaveric cut through a left middle ear (*ME*), showing the bony Eustachian tube (*Pr*) and the canal of tensor tympani muscle (*asterisk*), the isthmus (*I*), the cartilaginous Eustachian tube (*ET*), and its inferiorly related levator veli palatini muscle (*LVP*). The superior wall of the bony Eustachian tube is formed by the tegmen tubari

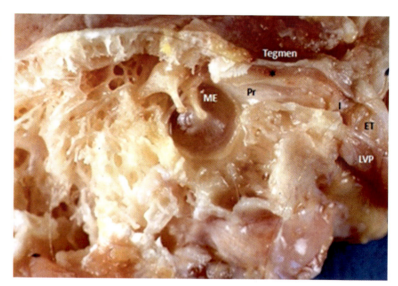

Fig. 7.9 (**a**) Transversal computed tomographic view of a right ear. Eustachian tube (*white arrow heads*), surrounded by numerous aerated cells (*white arrows*); *ICA* internal carotid artery. (**b**) Computed tomograpic reconstruction perpendicular to the Eustachian tube (*) showing an air cell opened into the Eustachian tube (*arrow*); TTM (*arrowhead*)

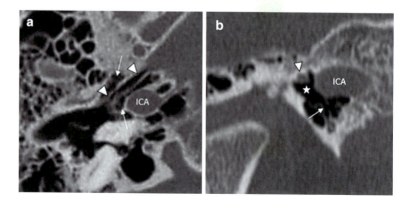

7.2.2   The Junctional Segment

The cartilaginous and bony portions of the ET are joined at a bottleneck area, the junctional segment of the ET.

This segment is 2 mm in height and 1 mm wide. It lies between the carotid canal medially and the temporomandibular joint and foramen spinosum with the middle meningeal artery laterally (Figs. 7.7).

Due to its reduced caliber, this segment plays a protective role for the middle ear against recurrent otitis media in preventing naso-pharyngeal secretions to enter the middle ear cavity.

7.2.3   The Fibrocartilaginous Tube

The fibrocartilaginous portion of the ET is 20–24 mm long; it extends along the base of the skull from its junction with the bony portion of the tube until the medial pterygoid plate. Posteriorly this part of the ET extends about 3 mm into the bony part and is firmly attached to it by fibrous bands [17–19]. It is angled 30°–40° to the transverse plane and 45° to the sagittal plane of the base of the skull [9]. The fibrocartilaginous part is loosely attached at this level in the sphenoid sulcus (sulcus tubae) between the greater wing of the sphenoid bone and the petrous portion of the temporal bone (Fig. 7.10).

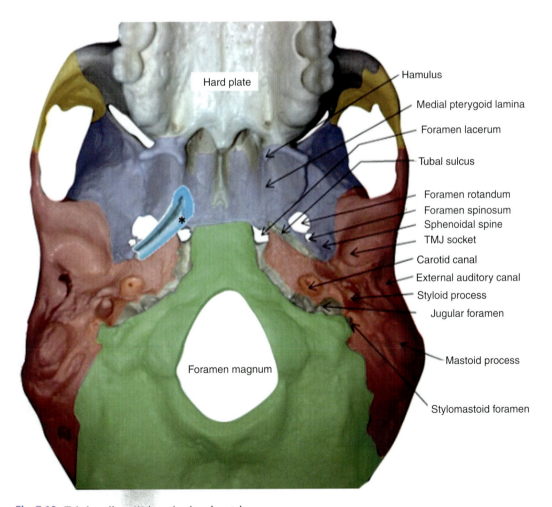

Fig. 7.10 Tubal cartilage (*) insertion in sulcus tubae

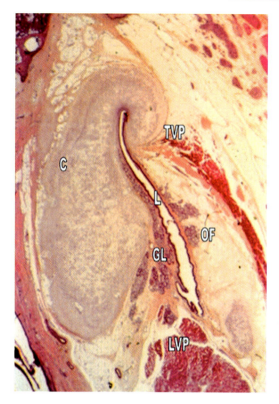

Fig. 7.11 Midcartilaginous portion of a normal left Eustachian tube of an adult temporal bone specimen. *C* cartilage, *L* lumen, *GL* submucosal glands, *LVP* levator veli palatini muscle, *TVP* tensor veli palatini muscle, *OF* Ostmann's fat pad (Courtesy of I. Sando, MD) (Reproduced with permission from Eustachian tube: structure, Function, Role in otitis media, by Charles D. Bluestone. pmph-usa.com)

The nasopharyngeal end of the tubal cartilage crosses the superior border of the superior pharyngeal constrictor muscle to enter the nasopharynx; it is tightly fixed by a broad attachment to a tubercle on the posterior edge of the medial pterygoid plate [15].

The fibrocartilaginous tube is composed of two components: the cartilaginous part, the major component that is completed laterally, and inferiorly by the fibromembranous part (Fig. 7.11).

7.2.3.1 The Cartilaginous Part

The cartilaginous portion of the ET is composed of one piece of cartilage that is shaped like a triangle at the top rear with a lower concavity. The apex or lateral end of the cartilaginous part

joins the bony portion at the isthmus; the wider medial end lies under the mucosa of the nasopharynx.

The tubal cartilage is an elastic cartilage and has an inverted J shape in cross section. It is composed of a short lateral lamina, an elongated medial lamina, and a hinge at the junction of the two laminas.

The lateral lamina has a constant height. However, the medial lamina starts as a short structure of 9 mm of height at the isthmus to increase rapidly to 13 mm just posterior and lateral to the attachment of the cartilage to the medial pterygoid plate [15]. The hinge portion, rich in elastin, serves to return the lateral lamina to its original position after active opening of the tube by TVP muscle contraction.

To form a tube, the cartilaginous portion is completed laterally and inferiorly by a veiled membrane, the fibrous part of the tube or fibrous wall (Fig. 7.11).

7.2.3.2 The Fibrous Part

The fibrous part represents the lateral and the inferior walls of the fibrocartilaginous ET. It is thick and resistant and called the *salpingopharyngeus fascia of Tröltsch*. Laterally, it serves as the site of insertion of the TVP muscle. The lateral part of the fascia of Tröltsch is inserted to the base of skull at the petrosphenoid suture (Proctor ligament) close to the foramen spinosum, foramen ovale, and the base of the pterygoid process laterally (see Fig. 7.10).

The medial part of the fascia of Tröltsch is anchored superiorly to the inferior curvature of the lateral lamina of the tubal cartilage. The region between the fascia and ET mucosa is occupied by a glandular tissue anteriorly and adipose tissue posteriorly. Thus, it is presumed that the forces developed by the TVP would pass to the lateral lamina of the cartilage rather than to the submucosa of the lumen to insure the opening of the tube.

7.2.3.3 Ostmann's Fat Pad

Ostmann's fat pad is a lympho-adipose body, situated around the pharyngeal end in the inferolateral aspect of the anterior part of the ET. It occupies the space between the ET proper and the TVP muscle (Fig. 7.11).

It is thought to represent an important contributing factor in closing the tube. It contributes to the protection of the ET and the middle ear from reflux of nasopharyngeal secretions. In malnourished persons this pad of fat is lost causing patulous ET.

Ostmann's fat pad increases in volume during childhood, being most voluminous in adults, and regresses in the elderly.

7.2.4 The Pharyngeal End

The pharyngeal end of the ET passes above the superior constrictor muscle through the sinus of Morgani to lay under the mucosa of the nasopharynx. The pharyngeal orifice lies approximately at the posterior level of the vomer, about 1.25 cm behind the posterior end of the inferior turbinate and approximately 2 cm above the plane of the hard palate [9].

The pharyngeal orifice is triangular in shape with an inferior base; it measures 8–10 mm in height and 3–5 mm in width (Figs. 7.6 and 7.12). The pharyngeal orifice is closed at rest and becomes elliptical or triangular with a superior apex during opening.

Its anterolateral border is a vertical prominent crease, called the salpingopalatine crease. It corresponds to the lateral plate of the tubal cartilage and the TVP muscle. The posteromedial border is prominent and corresponds to the medial lamella of the tubal cartilage pressing against the nasopharyngeal mucosa; this prominent surelevation of the mucosa is called the *torus tubari* (Fig. 7.12). The torus tubari thickness is of 10–15 mm [15]. The mucosa of the torus tubari is rich in glands and lymphoid tissue forming the *tonsil of Gerlach*. The inferior border of the pharyngeal orifice is bounded by the levator veli palatini muscle.

Just medial and behind the torus tubari there is a recess called the *fossa of Rosenmüller*, which is a triangular recess of about 1.5 cm deep. Its apex is in close relationship with the carotid canal, and its base is closely related to

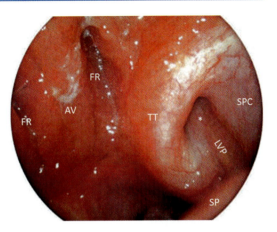

Fig. 7.12 Endoscopic view of left pharyngeal orifice. *FR* fossa of Rosenmuller, *AV* adenoid vegetation, *TT* torus tubari, *SPC*, salpingopalatine crease containing levator veli palatini muscle, *LVP* levator veli palatini muscle in the floor of the Eustachian tube, *SP* soft palate, * Eustachian tube lumen

the skull base with the foramen lacerum lying medially. Adenoid tissues usually extend into this recess giving soft tissue support to the ET (Fig. 7.12).

7.2.5 Muscles of the Eustachian Tube

Four muscles are associated with the ET: the tensor veli palatini (TVP), the levator veli palatini (LVP), the salpingopharyngeus, and the tensor tympani muscle.

ET is closed at rest and opens during swallowing or yawning. Active opening of the ET is induced by TVP muscle contraction [20–22]. Closure of the tube is a passive phenomenon and is not the result of a muscular contraction. It takes place secondarily to the passive reapproximation of the tubal walls by extrinsic forces exerted by the surrounding deformed tissues and also by the recoil of elastic fibers of the hinge portion [15].

7.2.5.1 Tensor Veli Palatini (TVP) Muscle

The TVP muscle is composed of two distinct bundles of muscle fibers: the lateral (superficial) and the medial (deep) bundle that are separated by a fibroelastic layer (Fig. 7.13).

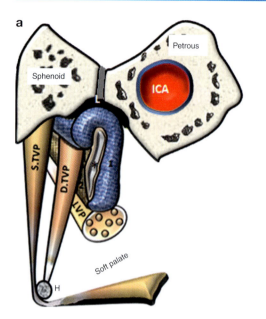 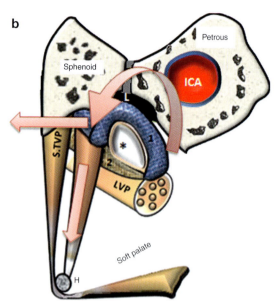

Fig. 7.13 Schematic representation of paratubal muscles and the action of tensor veli patine muscle. (**a**) During relaxation; (**b**) during contraction. *S.TVP* superficial bundle of tensor veli palatine muscle, medial bundle of *DTVP* deep bundle of tensor veli palatine muscle, *LVP* levator veli palatine muscle, *L* tubal ligament, *1* tubal cartilage, *2* tubal fibrous membrane, * tubal lumen, *H* hammulus, *ICA* internal carotid artery

The Lateral Bundle

The lateral bundle is not related to the ET function. It has an inverted triangular shape with a superior base and an inferior apex. It starts superiorly at the scaphoid fossa of the sphenoid bone lateral to the ET cartilage. Then, it descends anteriorly, laterally, and inferiorly to converge in a tendon that rounds the hamular process of the medial pterygoid lamina. From the hamular process it progresses to insert into the posterior border of the hard palate and into the palatine aponeurosis [15].

The lateral bundle of the TVP muscle ensures the tension of the soft palate.

The Medial Bundle

The medial bundle, also called the dilator tube muscle, has its superior origin in the posterior half of the lateral lamina of the cartilaginous ET. Its fibers descend sharply and converge in a tendon that inserts on the hamular process of the medial pterygoid plate.

The medial bundle is responsible for the active dilatation of the fibrocartilaginous tube by inferolateral displacement of its membranous wall [23–25].

Secondary attachments of the medial bundle are present sometimes at the maxillary tuberosity and the palatoglossal arch. These insertions suggest that even if the hamulus is in-fractured during cleft palate surgery, the TVP function could be maintained by preserving its maxillary insertion [26].

Both bundles are innervated by the mandibular nerve (V3).

7.2.5.2 The Levator Veli Palatini (LVP) Muscle (Fig. 7.13)

The LVP muscle arises from the inferior aspect of the petrous apex of the temporal bone. Its rounded body passes inferomedially, paralleling and lying beneath the floor of the fibrocartilaginous tube lumen. The fibers of this muscle insert by fanning out and blending with the dorsal surface of the soft palate [9, 17].

The LVP muscle is related to the tube only by a loose connective tissue [20, 27].

It is essentially a muscle serving the soft palate, but it could also support the ET function by elevating the medial lamina of the cartilage at the pharyngeal orifice [19, 28]. In addition, being located inferolaterally to the ET and with its large cross-sectional area in this portion, the LVP may be related to the pumping clearance (drainage) function of the tube in such a way that the distal end of the tube closes first followed progressively towards the pharyngeal orifice, thus pumping out the middle ear secretions [29].

The levator veli palatini is innervated by the glossopharyngeal nerve (IX).

7.2.5.3 The Salpingopharyngeal Muscle

The salpingopharyngeal muscle arises from the medial and inferior borders of the tubal cartilage via slips of muscular and tendinous fibers. Then the muscle courses inferoposteriorly to blend with the mass of the palatopharyngeal muscle. The salpingopharyngeal muscle is not involved in the function of the ET. It is innervated by the glossopharyngeal nerve IX [9, 27].

7.2.5.4 The Tensor Tympani Muscle

The tensor tympani muscle arises from the superior surface of the cartilaginous part of the auditory tube, the greater wing of the sphenoid, and the petrous part of the temporal bone. The muscle passes posterolaterally and always superiorly to the ET in its bony semicanal to the cochleariform process on the medial wall of the middle ear. Its tendon hooks around the cochleariform process to run laterally and insert into the medial aspect of the neck of the malleus. Contraction of the tensor tympani pulls the eardrum medially and restricts its mobility. Thus, sound transmission through the middle ear is attenuated when the tensor tympani is contracted. It is innervated by a branch of the mandibular nerve V3.

7.2.6 Eustachian Tube Mucosa

At the tympanic orifice of the ET, the lumen is of 2 mm in height and 5 mm in width. From the isthmus downwards, the lumen expands continuously to become about 8–10 mm in height and 1–2 mm in width at its pharyngeal orifice.

The lumen is lined by a pseudostratified, columnar epithelium of a ciliated type, which sweeps material from the middle ear to the nasopharynx. The mucosa is continuous with the lining of the tympanic cavity at its distal end, as it is with the nasopharynx at its proximal end. Associated with these ciliated epithelial cells are the goblet cells figuring about 20 % of the cell population [30, 31].

The floor mucosa of the tube contains numerous goblet cells, copious ciliated cells, and glands [31, 32]. The roof mucosa of the tube has sparse goblet cells and cuboidal ciliated cells without seromucous glands.

Therefore, we can recognize two different morpho-functional corridors in the ET lumen:
1. Superior corridor: the roof for the ventilation function
2. Inferior corridor: the floor with its mucociliary clearance function

7.2.7 Eustachian Tube Blood Vessels

The arterial blood supply of the ET is derived from the ascending pharyngeal and middle meningeal arteries. The venous drainage is carried to the pharyngeal and pterygoid plexus of veins. The lymphatic chains drain into the retropharyngeal lymph nodes.

7.2.8 Eustachian Tube Nerves

The ostium and the cartilagenous portion of the ET are innervated by the pharyngeal branch of the sphenopalatine ganglion deriving from the maxillary nerve (V2).

The bony portion of the ET is innervated by the tympanic plexus deriving from the glossopharyngeal nerve (IX).

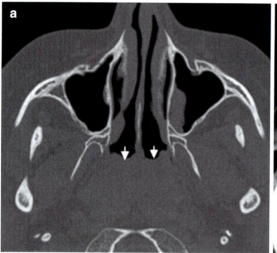 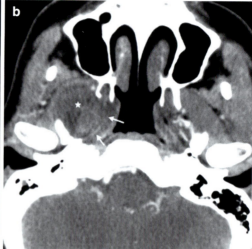

Fig. 7.14 (**a**) Transversal computed tomography of a 15-year-old boy with bilateral adhesive otitis media. Huge adenoid hypertrophy (*white arrows*) in the nasopharynx. (**b**) Transversal injected computed tomography of an adult showing a well-encapsulated globulous lesion (schwannoma) of the right infratemporal fossa (*), with a mass effect (*white arrows*) on the Eustachian tube

Clinical Application
Eustachian Tube Function

Although the osseous portion of the ET remains patent and is not dynamic, the cartilaginous portion of the ET is normally closed and opens only for brief periods of time. This situation blocks the nasopharyngeal secretions or a gastric reflux from entering into the middle ear as well as it prevents autophonia.

Brief intermittent periods of ET opening occur in normal individuals to insure middle ear ventilation. The ET opens 1.5 times every minute. Every opening lasts about 0.5 seconds [33]. These openings are the result of the contractions of TVP muscle.

In addition, the ET insures the function of the middle ear mucociliary clearance. The ciliated epithelial cells of the lumen floor provide a mucociliary "elevator" to push debris and secretions downwards from the ET into the nasopharynx.

Impairment of the tubal function can be divided into two main categories: *Eustachian tube dysfunction* when the tube does not open properly or *patulous* *Eustachian tube* when the tube remains inappropriately patent.

Eustachian Tube Dysfunction

ET dysfunction could be the result of mucosal inflammation with edema and obstruction, or anatomical extrinsic obstruction, or failure of dilatation from muscular problems causing dilatory dynamic dysfunction.

Dilatatory dynamic dysfunction of the ET is a strong contributor for ET disorders in infants [34, 35].

Anatomical extrinsic obstruction must always be ruled out. In children and adolescent, anatomical obstruction could be frequently due to adenoid hypertrophy. In adults presenting unilateral ET dysfunction, nasopharyngeal or infratemporal fossa tumors must be ruled out (Fig. 7.14).

Intrinsic blockage of the ET is more common than anatomical extrinsic obstruction. It is often the result of mucosal inflammation (mucosal disease), possibly due to allergies or laryngopharyngeal reflux. Tobacco use results in a loss of the

Table 7.1 Anatomical differences of the Eustachian tube between infants and adults

	Infant	Adult
Length (mm)	Approximately 15	Approximately 30
Cartilaginous portion	Less than 2/3 of the tube	2/3 of the tube
Bony portion	Relatively larger and wider than the adult	Relatively smaller
Pharyngeal orifice	About ½ that of the adult but similar width	Height 8 mm, width 2 mm
Angulation with respect to base of skull (°)	10	45
Tensor veli palatini muscle action	Less efficient	More efficient
Ostmann's pad fat	Less prominent	Prominent

normal ciliary clearance of the mucosa and causes frequently ET dysfunction.

Patulous Eustachian Tube

Patulous ET occurs when the ET tube remains patent for long periods of time beyond the normal brief interval of opening. This condition could be related to Ostmann's fat pad atrophy that may develop after substantial weight loss or post-pregnancy.

Patients with patulous ET typically complain of autophonia and aural fullness. When patients lie down, the symptoms usually abate due to venous engorgement of ET mucosa.

Infantile Eustachian Tube

The differences in the anatomy of the ET between infants and adults explain the functional differences that play an important role in the inflammatory pathology of the middle ear and their complications.

Dilatory dynamic dysfunction of the ET is a strong contributor for ET dysfunction in infants. In infants, the shallow tubal angle affects adversely the muscle vector of the TVP, which in addition to the highly compliant tubal cartilage leads to a failure of active opening of ET by TVP muscle contraction [34, 35].

Changes in the tubal angle and the cartilage strength until adulthood are responsible for more efficient active opening of the ET, improved protective role and an improved clearance function (Fig. 7.5 and Table 7.1).

References

1. Proctor B. Embryology and anatomy of the Eustachian tube. Arch Otolaryngol. 1967;86:503–26.
2. Swarts JD, Rood SR, Doyle WJ. Fetal development of the auditory tube and paratubal musculature. Cleft Palate J. 1986;23:289–311.
3. Wolff D. The microscopic anatomy of the Eustachian tube. Ann Otol Rhinol Laryngol. 1934;43:483.
4. Tos M. Growth of the fetal Eustachian tube and its dimensions. Arch Klin Exp Ohren Nasen Kehlkopfheilkd. 1971;198:177–86.
5. Sadler-Kimes D, Siegel MI, Todhunter JS. Age-related morphologic differences in the components of the Eustachian tube/middle-ear system. Ann Otol Rhinol Laryngol. 1989;98:854–8.
6. Siegel MI, Cantekin EI, Todhunter JS, Sadler-Kimes D. Aspect ratio as a descriptor of Eustachian tube cartilage shape. Ann Otol Rhinol Laryngol. 1988;97 Suppl 133:16–7.
7. Siegel MI, Sadler-Kimes D, Todhunter JS. ET cartilage shape as a factor in the epidemiology of otitis media. In: Lim DJ, Bluestone CD, Klein JO, Nelson JD, editors. Recent advances in otitis media: proceedings of the Fourth International Symposium. Burlington: BC Decker; 1988. p. 114–7.
8. Ishijima K, Sando I, Balaban C, Suzuki C, Takasaki K. Length of the Eustachian tube and its postnatal development: computer-aided three dimensional reconstruction and measurement study. Ann Otol Rhinol Laryngol. 2000;109:542–8.
9. Graves GO, Edwards LF. The Eustachian tube: review of its descriptive, microscopic, topographic, and clinical anatomy. Arch Otolaryngol. 1944;39:359–97.
10. Matsune S, Sando I, Takahashi H. Comparative study of elastic at the hinge portion of Eustachian tube cartilage in normal and cleft palate individuals. In: Lim DJ, Bluestone CD, Klein JO, et al., editors. Recent advances in otitis media: proceedings of the Fifth International Symposium. Burlington: BC Decker; 1993. p. 4–6.
11. Suzuki C, Balaban CD, Sando I, et al. Postnatal development of Eustachian tube: a computer-aided 3-D reconstruction and measurement study. Acta Otolaryngol (Stockh). 1998;118:837–43.

12. Orita Y, Sando I, Hasebe S, Miura M. Postnatal change on the location of Ostmann's fatty tissue in the region lateral to Eustachian tube. Int J Pediatr Otorhinolaryngol. 2003;67:1105–12.

13. Prades JM, Dumollard JM, Calloc'h F, Merzougui N, Veyret C, Martin C. Descriptive anatomy of the human auditory tube. Surg Radiol Anat. 1998;20(5):335–40.

14. Sudo M, Sando I, Ikui A, Suzuki C. Narrowest (isthmus) portion of Eustachian tube: a computer-aided three-dimensional reconstruction and measurement study. Ann Otol Rhinol Laryngol. 1997;106:583–8.

15. Bluestone CD, Bluestone MB, Coulter J. Eustachian tube: structure, function, role in otitis media. Hamilton/Lewiston: BC Decker; 2005. p. 25–50.

16. Jen A, Sanelli PC, Banthia V, et al. Relationship of petrous temporal bone pneumatization to the Eustachian tube lumen. Laryngoscope. 2004;114:656–60.

17. Bryant WS. The Eustachian tube: its anatomy and its movement: with a description of the cartilages, muscles, fasciae, and the fossa of Rosenmüller. Med Rec. 1907;71:931.

18. Rood SR, Doyle WJ. The nasopharyngeal orifice of the auditory tube: implications for tubal dynamics anatomy. Cleft Palate J. 1982;19:119–28.

19. Swarts JD, Rood SR. The morphometry and three-dimensional structure of the adult Eustachian tube: implications for function. Cleft Palate J. 1990;27: 374–81.

20. Rich AR. A physiological study of the Eustachian tube and its related muscles. Bull Johns Hopkins Hosp. 1920;31:3005–10.

21. Cantekin EI, Doyle WJ, Reichert TJ, et al. Dilation of the Eustachian tube by electrical stimulation of the mandibular nerve. Ann Otol Rhinol Laryngol. 1979;88:40–51.

22. Honjo I, Okazaki N, Kumazawa T. Experimental study of the Eustachian tube function with regard to its related muscles. Acta Otolaryngol (Stockh). 1979;87:84–9.

23. Simkins C. Functional anatomy of the Eustachian tube. Arch Otolaryngol. 1943;38:476.

24. Goss C, editor. Gray's anatomy of the human body. Philadelphia: Lea & Febiger; 1967.

25. Canalis RF. Valsalva's contribution to otology. Am J Otolaryngol. 1990;11:420–7.

26. Abe M, Murakami G, Noguchi M, et al. Variations in the tensor veli palatine muscle with special reference to its origin and insertion. Cleft Palate Craniofac J. 2004;41:474–84.

27. McMyn JK. The anatomy of the salpingopharyngeus muscle. J Laryngol Otol. 1940;55:1–22.

28. Sudo M, Sando I, Suzuki C. Three dimensional reconstruction and measurement of human Eustachian tube structures: a hypothesis of Eustachian tube function. Ann Otol Rhinol Laryngol. 1998;107: 547–54.

29. Ishijima K, Sando I, Miura M, et al. Postnatal development of static volume of the Eustachian tube lumen. Ann Otol Rhinol Laryngol. 2002;111:832–5.

30. Lim DJ. Functional morphology of the tubotympanum. Acta Otolaryngol (Stockh). 1984;98 Suppl 414: 13–8.

31. Tos M, Bak-Pedersen K. Goblet cell population in the normal middle ear and Eustachian tube of children and adults. Ann Otol Rhinol Laryngol. 1976;85 Suppl 25:44–50.

32. Sando I, Takahashi H, Matsune S, Aoki H. Localization of function in the Eustachian tube: a hypothesis. Ann Otol Rhinol Laryngol. 1993;103:311–4.

33. Mondain M, Vidal D, Bouhanna S. Uziel, Monitoring Eustachian tube opening: Preliminary results in normal subjects. Laryngoscope. 1997;107:1414–9.

34. Bylander A, Tjernstrom O, Ivarsson A. Pressure opening and closing functions of the Eustachian tube by inflation and deflation in children and adults with normal ears. Acta Otolaryngol (Stockh). 1983;96: 255–68.

35. Bylander A, Tjernstrom O. Changes in Eustachian tube function with age in children with normal ears: a longitudinal study. Acta Otolaryngol (Stockh). 1983;96:467–77.

Index

Printing and Binding: Stürtz GmbH, Würzburg